W9-DGS-062

**Making
Health
Education
Work**

Making Health Education Work

Health education
in health program development,
with primary attention on programming
for low-income and minority groups

Publisher:
American Public Health Association
1015 Eighteenth Street, N.W.
Washington, D.C. 20036

Printed in the United States of America

Library of Congress Catalog Number: 76-26205
International Standard Book Number: 0-87553-080-X

July, 1976

Library of Congress Cataloging in Publication Data

Main entry under title:

Making health education work.

   Foreword signed: Jeannette Simmons, chairperson/editor.
   Bibliography: p.
   1. Health education. 2. Poor--Health and hygiene. 3. Minorities--Health and hygiene. I. Simmons, Jeannette. II. American Public Health Association. [DNLM: 1. Health education--Congresses. 2. Poverty--Congresses. 3. Minority groups--Congresses. WA590 M235 1974-75]
RA440.5.M32 362.1 76-26205
ISBN 0-87553-080-X

The research encompassed in this text was funded under a grant by The Upjohn Company to the Health Education Research Council, Inc. The workshop program, the National Conference on Consumer Health Education and the preparation of the text were supervised by an Advisory Committee of members nominated by the American Public Health Association and The Society for Public Health Education.

Foreword

Within these pages are assembled ideas, experience and advice drawn from over 100 health education programs. Seventeen of them were examined in fine detail at three regional workshops. The major issues arising out of these studies were then further reviewed by top experts in health-related fields, who added their own experience and interpretation at the National Conference on Consumer Health Education in October, 1974.

Publication of the work of this Project has a double purpose: (1) to help those already busy carrying out health education programs, and (2) to help the many others who, in the inevitable course of health care progress, will soon become involved with health education—administering it, paying for it, or using it.

The material presented was developed over the past three years under the guidance of a General Advisory Committee, whose members were appointed by the Health Education Section of the American Public Health Association and the Society for Public Health Education.

The Committee became involved in this effort as a response to a request to *SOPHE* and *APHA* by *The Upjohn Company*, asking how Upjohn could best contribute to the health education of low-income and minority consumers. In the first year, the Committee provided guidance for the development of a consumer education program in the Family Health Center in Kalamazoo, Michigan's Northside neighborhood. This health education program was primarily supported by Upjohn.

In the second year, the Committee's functions were broadened to the approaches covered—documenting and evaluating the experiences of many practitioners in a variety of health settings. Their diverse educational approaches are used to illustrate common elements in the educational process as they apply to the health field.

Appreciation is due the many individuals and organizations whose contributions made this Project possible. Members of the General Advisory Committee often made personal and professional sacrifices to devote the needed time to many aspects of the endeavor. A special note of thanks also goes to those individuals who contributed so freely of their time and thought by providing programs for review, attending workshops and participating in the National Conference. The latter individuals are identified in the Appendix.

The Upjohn Company management deserves our profound gratitude for providing financial support for the Project, initiating action for this effort, patience in working with the Committee, and foresight in addressing one of the major problems facing society: How to improve the quality of life for those who are deprived.

Finally, special acknowledgement is given to Cecilia Conrath Doak, Anna Skiff and Edward E. Greene for their untiring assistance in the task of selecting and organizing the material presented in this report. The exhaustive task as recorder for the three workshops was undertaken by Daniel Sullivan.

The completion of a collaborative effort of this sort produces mixed feelings of satisfaction and relief and a grave concern that some crucial contribution has been overlooked. The Committee members trust this Supplement will be a useful resource for health workers and community groups as they review, refine and/or initiate an educational approach in some aspect of their program.

Jeannette Simmons, D.Sc.
Chairperson/Editor

Table of Contents

Health Education Project
General Advisory Committee

Dr. Jeannette Simmons, Committee Chairman
Associate Professor, Harvard School of Public
  Health
Harvard University, Boston, MA

Mr. Kenneth Alston
Community Health Service Dept. HEW
Philadelphia, PA

Mr. Caesar Branchini
Executive Assistant, Blue Cross & Blue Shield of
  Greater NY
New York, NY

Dr. Donald A. Campbell
Asst. Prof. of Dept. of Preventive Medicine
Ohio State University, Columbus, OH

Mrs. Cecilia Conrath Doak
Potomac, MD

Mr. Daniel Sullivan
Editor/Publisher
Health Education Report
Ojai, CA

Dr. Courtney Wood,
Associate Professor of Community Medicine, Mt.
Sinai School of Medicine, New York, NY
Associate Chief of Staff for Allied Health & Education
Bronx Veterans Administration Hospital
Bronx, NY

Project Coordinator
Ms. Anna Skiff
USPHS Hospital, Staten Island, NY

Project Liaison
Mr. Richard Y. St. John
The Upjohn Company
Kalamazoo, MI

I. Introduction

The information assembled here represents the first effort to present an overall picture of how health education principles were applied in the past decade to health programs serving low-income and minority groups. It includes suggestions for strengthening educational efforts, and it points up deficiencies which must be overcome if education is to realize its potential value in the health system.

The Project sought information about the planning, organization, operation and management of learning experiences directed toward the improved health behavior of poor people. It also focused on determining what programs have done to determine the effectiveness of the educational efforts. The Committee based its definition of health education on that arrived at by the Joint Committee on Health Education Terminology.*

In considering the role of health education in

---

* This definition comes from the Health Education monograph #33, 1973, New Definitions, prepared by the Joint Committee on Health Education Terminology. The definition reads: "A process with intellectual, psychological, and social dimensions relating to activities which increase the abilities of people to make informed decisions affecting their personal, family, and community well-being. This process, based on scientific principles, facilitates learning and behavioral change in both health personnel and consumers, including children and youth."

the planning of health programs, members of the Health Education Project Advisory Committee recognized there are many opportunities for people to learn about health in the course of a health program or while receiving some specific kind of health care. Health education was viewed as being potentially a part of all health programs which require voluntary action by an individual, a family or a community.

The Committee defined the educational process as including these considerations:

A. Personal and situational factors create and influence the behavior patterns that already exist.

B. The "learner" must be involved in defining his own goals and actions and must evolve a way of achieving them within his own framework of values, beliefs, and resources.

C. Many experiences, both positive and negative, have an impact on what an individual, a group, or a community thinks, feels, and does about health.

D. Changes in behavior, to be long-lasting and practiced regularly, must be self-imposed; they cannot be administratively ordered. The behavior must be integrated into the individual's life patterning.

E. All educational efforts are based on the promotion of a sense of individual identity, dignity, and responsibility, as well as community solidarity.

F. The promotion of health action must be in keeping with the services and resources available, so that false expectations and frustrations will not develop.

Purpose of Project

The Project has looked at what is involved in using any of a variety of educational opportunities as a way to improve health care, especially of low-income or minority groups. There are valuable lessons in the largely unpublished experience of people who, during the past decade, have carried on educational programs. The excitement and frenzied bandwagon activity of the '60's to develop health services and programs for the underserved, poor and disenfranchised slowed to the pace of survival tactics in the early '70's. Now the focus has shifted to evaluating what can be done within the limited financial and manpower sources which most health education programs have available.

At this stage of stock-taking, there is a need to examine the special benefits that have been gained through past efforts. In this way the education methods which have proved effective with minority groups can become more widely accepted as standard operating procedures.

The Committee members determined there was a need to delineate more precisely the elements that make a health education program successful or unsuccessful, and they felt that to do this, further information was needed.

Information Collection Methods

To gather information the Committee issued a broad call throughout the nation for examples from all types of settings that might show how health education could be used, both to improve consumer health directly and also to achieve better use of existing health services. The Committee received over 100 written reports of health education programs from 36 states.

Material flowed in from individuals as well as voluntary health agencies, state and local health departments, hospitals, universities, medical centers, health care corporations, neighborhood health centers, and from health components of Model Cities programs. The groups served included Black, Spanish-speaking, Asian, American Indian, Eskimo and heterogeneous populations. Common to all was an attempt to find more effective ways to reach people who were poorly served by existing health programs.

The programs submitted often had successes in one or more aspects of the educational process, as well as failures in others. The Committee selected for further documentation a variety of programs which illustrate various elements in the educational process, rather than selecting only those with major accomplishments or for "excellence."

An in-depth analysis was made of the "life-histories" of 17 programs at workshops held during April and May, 1974, in New York, San Francisco, and Columbus, Ohio. The goals, methods and results of the 17 were studied, with the intent of probing beyond written reports, which are apt to omit or gloss over important ideas in program development that would be helpful to someone just beginning a program. Staff members of the various projects all followed the same outline in describing their activities. (A full example is presented in the Appendix.) They were then "de-briefed" by other workshop participants and members of the Advisory Committee.

Following the workshops, a three-day National Conference was held in October 1974, to familiarize people responsible for the management of health education and health delivery systems with the opportunities and constraints in consumer health education. Three critical issues revealed by the previous workshop discussions and project analyses were examined. They were:

A. Social and organizational barriers to consumer involvement.
B. Gaining and maintaining support for programs.
C. Assessing accomplishment.

The total effort brought together many imaginative and resourceful persons. They generated an excitement about the potential contribution that health education can make to the accessibility and acceptibility of health services for consumers.

This report contains the results of the discussions and project analyses. It is organized to suggest a systematic way of dealing with the major components of education for health.

Timeliness and Importance of Project

Why is it important to consider changing traditional understandings and attitudes about health education?

● There is a growing desire on the part of consumers to learn more about what constitutes good health care.

● The Neighborhood and Family Health Center movements seek to build stronger bonds with the people they serve by using community residents as health workers; this creates new possibilities for education.

• Some organizations that provide health care want to develop greater self-reliance among consumers in managing their own health problems, both as a way to keep costs down and as an expression of human rights.

Steps[1] taken recently by the legislative and the health community also highlight health education:

• Educational services must be provided by Health Maintenance Organizations which receive Federal funding.

• Health insurance carriers have taken steps to include payment for patient education in their coverage.

• "Quality of care" assessments bring out the need for greater attention to education as a way to prevent and cope with an illness.

As a result of these early pressures for more health education many people are looking for help in designing and carrying out educational programs. The report describes and illustrates important things to consider in such endeavors—all tempered by the insights gained in the workshops and the National Conference.

The findings of the Project are presented in the report in a sequence which has been determined to be the pathway that most local level practitioners follow in coping with the requirements of their own programs. It became apparent from program contributors that few programs spring into existence full-blown according to a pre-set plan. One seldom begins neatly and rationally, but instead usually finds oneself caught up in the flow of events. However, even in these circumstances, examples were found where it was possible to take into account the conflicting needs and pressures and still construct a sound program.

Programs Reviewed at the Workshops

Titles and abbreviated descriptions of the 17 projects studied in the workshops are given here as an aid to readers, who will find references to many of these projects in the text. Those wishing to request further information (if available) about a project may write to the name and address provided in the appendix under "Workshop Participants."

New York State Health Guides Project—A program that uses neighborhood outreach workers to motivate people in the inner city to support and participate in specific environmental health campaigns. Illustrations of how the guides contribute were obtained from several communities.

Project Enable—A nationwide training program, carried out jointly by three social agencies using parent group education to show disadvantaged parents how to cope with their problems more effectively; 99 agencies in 62 communities participated.

Consumer Education in Comprehensive Health Planning—A Columbia University effort, which provided seven courses and three leadership training sessions to help central Harlem residents prepare for membership on health committees and boards. The courses were designed to help consumers express community health needs, increase their understanding of administrative problems, and develop participation skills related to their roles in decision-making bodies.

Roosevelt Hospital (N.Y.C.) Health Education Project—Based in the Dept. of Pediatrics, this educational program seeks to improve the health status of users of the Children and Youth clinic and to find effective ways to involve members of the community in community education. The project is also interested in measuring the savings which can be derived by correcting inapropriate use of the clinic by both consumers and staff.

University of Maryland's Cooperative Extension Service Health Education Project—Developed as part of a national effort to combine with medical delivery systems the community outreach networks (Extension Services) of Land Grant Institutions with medical delivery systems. This project focused on the development of good preventive health practices and leadership abilities in teenagers.

VISTA Bi-Lingual Health Aides—The Hawaii State Department of Health extended the work of its Health Education Office by supporting the use of bi-lingual volunteer health aides through the VISTA program. The aides are used to assist newly-arriving immigrants with problems relating to tuberculosis and help them gain access to community health services.

IPHS Indian Health Service Utilization of Community Health Representatives—The program has been developed to assist tribal councils in employing tribal people as trained community health representatives within each community. Two tribal groups under the Portland, Ore., area Indian Health Office were used to illustrate how this program works at the community level.

Ventura County (Calif.) Health Services Delivery System—This project illustrates a community-wide effort involving consumers and health care providers from health and health-related agencies in the development of health care referral centers. The referral system uses trained volunteers, outreach workers and triage nurses to provide health consumers with access to services and education.

The McGrath Project (Alaska)—A project in which health educators and nurses, traveling to villages by plane, boat or dog team, demonstrated that increased health education, combined with a modest increase in health care, could make a significant dent in the high incidence of acute and chronic respiratory and ear disease in the native communities.

Texas Consumer Participation in Health Planning—Staff and associates of the American Friends Service Committee bridged the communications gap between the dominant and the low-income segments of communities, showing that poor Chicano and other low-income individuals can become effective participants in analyzing the health problems of their communities, setting priorities of need and developing plans to meet these needs.

Michigan Consumer Support Group—This project

researched the changes which could be achieved in consumer participation in comprehensive health planning when consumers were provided training in group problem-solving. The consumers were provided with opportunities to gain needed information, learn how to use their power and become effective participants in the health care system.

This was accomplished by creating a self-sustaining and autonomous group of consumers.

The Forty Family Pilot Study—Middle-income volunteer families worked one-on-one with 40 low-income families in Indiana, using outreach health aides and State Board of Health education materials. They increased nutritional awareness, the use of medical resources, and, through educational and occupational assistance, brought about an average 38 percent increase in family income in the first year.

Full Time Practical Nursing Program in the Evening for New Professionals—The Atlanta (Ga.) Southside Comprehensive Health Center developed a 12-month training program which gave many of its lowest-paid employees a credentialed and marketable skill as practical nurses.

Better Outpatient Health Care Through Improved Consumer Education—The Martland Hospital, Newark, N.J., brought together consumers, hospital staffs and staffs from community agencies to plan ways of improving the utilization of an outpatient department. They jointly developed videotapes and other health education materials to increase the consumers' understanding of health problems and services. They also effected changes in the delivery system.

Indian Health Service Community Health Aide Training Program—This program collected data on how the health status of Alaskan natives was raised by making the community health aide a primary health care provider and a positive influence in prevention of health problems.

Bynum Mill Neighborhood Project—This illustrates the work of the District Health Department of Chatham County, N.C., in its efforts to improve or stabilize the health of a neighborhood by making health care and health education available and accessible in a manner acceptable to the residents.

Involving the Uninvolved in Cancer Prevention—The Los Angeles County Branch of the American Cancer Society worked with interested Mexican-American women in ways they themselves suggested, bringing about different types of programs and materials for cancer education.

REFERENCES

1. "An HMO shall encourage and actively provide for its members education services and education in the contribution each member can make to the maintenance of his own health," *P.L. 93-222.*

   "The Congress finds that the following deserve priority consideration in the formulation of a national policy and in the development and operation of Federal, State and area health planning resources development . . . the development of effective methods for educating the general public on proper personal health care and methods for effective use of available health services." *P.L. 93-641.*

   "The patient has the right to obtain from his physician complete current information concerning his diagnosis, treatment, and prognosis in terms the patient can reasonably be expected to understand." *Patient's Bill of Rights—American Hospital Assoc., 1972.*

"The AMA supports the concept of Indian self-determination as the strength of successful Indian programs and recognizes that acceptable solution to Indian health problems can result only when the program and project beneficiaries have an initial and continued major contribution in planning and program operation." Recommendation adopted by the *AMA House of Delegates, December, 1973.*

"A major innovation of the Neighborhood Health Center is the chance it offers for the direct involvement of the people served." *Economic Opportunity Act Amendments of 1967.*

II. Initiating a Health Education Program

This section deals with five findings from the Health Education Project which appear to affect the success of any health education program. The guidelines used by the Project Committee for in-depth studies of 17 projects and in the analyses of the discussion reflect accepted principles of health education developed over a long period of time. To relate these principles to the development and administration of a health program may provide fresh insight into ways of improving health behavior. The findings deal with:

- The origin of idea or need
- Time as a factor in building trust and credibility
- Consequences of early termination
- Ambiguity of data
- Relationships to non-health issues

Each of these findings will be discussed separately. Program descriptions in the Appendix amplify the points made here.

Origin of the Idea or Need

Tradition, logic, and textbooks all agree that those who are to benefit from a health education service—the target group—should be involved very early in the identification of need and in the determination of what actions should be undertaken. An examination of what *actually* happens under time, money, and staff constraints indicates that this early involvement occurs infrequently. The 17 programs and others analyzed proved to have a variety of origins:

- The interest of one individual . . . "Someone with power was interested."

- The pressures of society . . . "It became a responsibility of a lot of high-level agencies to find ways to improve conditions."

- The money was there . . "Many times the availability of funds brought about the initiation of a program."

- The response to needs identified by professionals . . . "The Commissioner of Health and others in Alaska were disturbed about the extraordinary incidence of chronic respiratory and ear disease in the native population. They promoted the project as an attempt to demonstrate whether or not increased health education, combined with a modest increase in treatment, could make a significant dent in the chronic ear and respiratory problems."

In actual fact, the program or project was seldom originated by members of the group served. Discussion revealed some of the reasons:

- "They didn't know there was anything they could do about it."

● "Sometimes they know there is a problem, but they are not in a position to do anything."

● "Anthropologists have found that people who are part of a community accept the fact that this is the way you live . . ."

What is crucial for a program to catch on and flourish is the sharing of ideas and plans as soon as possible with the community that is going to be affected. "They should learn how and why the professional community arrived at the conclusions they plan to implement."

If there is to be input from the consumer group served, the design of the program must be flexible enough to accommodate this input.

As Benjamin Paul[1] points out,

To work effectively with people, we must not only be able to see the world as they see it, but must understand the psychological and social functions performed in their practices and beliefs. These functions are not always evident to the people themselves."

Time constraints on a program must be dealt with. Questions asked often are: How much time is needed to get a program underway? How long must a program be in operation before results can be expected? Are there differences in the amount of time required to work with different cultural groups? What are the consequences of terminating a project prematurely?

Time as a Factor in Building Trust

The first question to be considered is how much time should be allowed for pre-planning. Among the 17 projects studied, six months was the shortest time spent in the pre-planning stage, and five years was the most extended period of time required.

Factors which influence the length of time it takes to get a program underway include:

- The number of people and agencies which must be involved—the greater the number, the longer the time.

- The experience of the funding agency. A long-established agency or funder has its guidelines set regarding program, while a new funder must create policies and evolve its approach while it is evaluating a particular request.

One project reported,

"Seven months were spent in planning and negotiating the contract. After it was awarded, an additional four months were required to accomplish local funding arrangements. During that period there were many meetings with the funders, many modifications of the original proposal, conferences, phone calls, and correspondence with people who were to be involved or who might expedite the process."

A shorter period of time elapses between the time funding is obtained and when the program addresses its objectives. No more than six months appears to be needed for this stage.

How long must a program be in operation before results can be expected? The data examined from the programs studied indicate that consumer education programs should be carried on for a minimum of three years and optimally for five years, so that enough time is available to build the relationships that are fundamental to successful intervention through education, and to conduct the activity itself.

Among the reasons cited for this amount of time to build trust were the following:

- A good period of time has to be spent with the health care providers and staff. As expressed within one project, "It takes a long time for a staff person to swallow the fact that a catastrophe will not occur if something happens they are not familiar with."

- "In some communities everyone has to discuss any idea that is proposed. This is a laborious process and can take a year. If you try to push, they'll dig in their feet and say 'Go somewhere else.'"

- "When you are putting something into the community that wasn't there before, you have to let people feel it out. A few brave souls will try it; the rest hang back to see the consequences. Things don't always get up and run the way you plan."

Are there differences in the amount of time

required to work with different cultural groups? Ethnic groups frequently do conceptualize time differently. Among Orientals, for example, the next month or two does not carry the same sense of urgency that project staff feel. They ask, "Why are you in such an all-fire hurry?"

The health care provider, having greater control over the program activities than the consumer, is in the best position to shorten the time period. For provider and consumer to work together effectively, the provider first must make sure of his own communications skills (1) by transmitting information in simple terms and adjusting to the culture of the consumer group, and (2) by encouraging and making use of the insights and creative responses that every group is capable of generating.

Adaptation to a new culture may be an unsettling experience for those who provide health care as well as for those who receive it. But the responsibility for developing the understanding rests with the providers, since this is the group introducing the changes.

In building credibility with the consumer group a certain sensitivity and self-awareness in providers was found to be important. For example, some workshop participants cited phrases that turn off minority people, such as, "Thanks for inviting me *down here*." Another expression sometimes used is "*you people*," which emphasizes the social distance between providers and consumers.

A community with divided leadership or a complex power structure may require a much longer time for the decision-making stages than a cohesive community. The community's past experience with other attempts at health education also will affect the amount of time required to build trust, depending on whether those experiences were good or bad. (Ways of dealing with this issue are discussed in Chapter IV, "Developing a Program.")

Consequences of Early Termination

What are the consequences of terminating a project prematurely? Several can be stated: (1) No valid conclusions can be drawn about either the success or failure of the approaches used; (2) substantial financial investment may be lost; (3) staff commitment may be destroyed and community confidence seriously eroded; (4) the resulting loss of community trust has the further effect of making it doubly difficult for any subsequent program to establish itself.

Equally disturbing as programs ended prematurely is the proliferation of "crash" campaigns labeled as education, which stir people into action without prior investigation of whether the community is capable of maintaining the new level of improved health change or service.

In describing some lessons learned in the 1960's, Eli Ginzberg[2] states:

> *"Almost by definition, a new social program is likely to be hobbled at first by the lack of knowledge and experience of those charged with its design and operation. A sensible public and its legislative representatives will allow time and resources for knowledge and experience to be accumulated. The required knowledge can be generated only by action, at least on an experimental scale. Moreover, a democracy has no option but to act as it learns."*

It is apparent that groups being served vary greatly in the way they view and act on health matters. Each group responds differently to its particular leadership, and each one attempts to retain the customs and beliefs associated with its ethnic background. Each of these factors influences the amount of time, manpower, and resources needed to get a project launched successfully.

Ambiguity of Data

All administrators and decision-makers seek data that are reliable (i.e., would turn out the same way if compiled a second time) and valid (i.e., measure what they are intended to measure). Yet it is difficult to attain these kinds of high-quality data when serving groups whose life style and perception of survival leads them to give whatever information they think the inquirer wants to hear.

The Project uncovered a number of examples of ambiguity in what one learns about a population. A few are cited here:

● Workers who had experience working with Chicanos stressed that most of the contemporary research on Chicanos is inaccurate and perpetuates stereotypes. They advise that one needs to distinguish clearly between Chicano cultural attributes, as expressed at all socio-economic levels by beliefs and practices, and those exhibited especially by people living in poverty. The barrios and colonias, groupings of Mexican-Americans and Chicano people, who are mostly low-income farm workers, may look the same to an outsider, but each has its own organizational pattern and set of dynamics.

- A staff of white professionals reported a major blunder in assuming that they should not offer the same background information to black professionals that was provided for other white resource people, in preparation for meeting with a black group. The training staff thought they would be imposing unreal (white) standards on the black speakers. This decision not only created distrust but also placed the black professionals at a disadvantage.

There are special problems in relying on verbal information. In low-income communities much information is transmitted by word of mouth—the grapevine. However, as the message goes through, it becomes distorted, so reliance only on this method may bring forth half-truths.

Many examples can be cited regarding the problems of obtaining consistent, reliable, and valid data. But what can be done about the situation as it exists? Probably the most important thing to realize is that data obtained from and about a target population are tentative. Time and resources must be provided for a periodic check on the reliability and validity of both the source and the information itself. To avoid future problems, several members of the group should be consulted to increase the likelihood that the information obtained will prove useful in deciding what to include or leave out of a training program.

To assume that attitudes or practices in a community are static is short-sighted and may result in expensive mistakes. It is better to question data about community power structure and look for changes, which may occur in subtle as well as overt ways. In this area it also is important to seek ways to validate information through written sources as well as through personal observations.

Relationships to Non-Health Issues

One of the dilemmas facing health professionals initiating a new health program is pressure to produce results within the time frame of the grant or the funding conditions. The need for time to prepare the community to accept a new program into its lives is commonly overlooked. The health worker often needs to help a consumer overcome a pressing personal problem before he or she is ready to act on a health condition.

One of the best ways to gain the acceptance of a group for your program is first to help individual members to solve their urgent personal problems. Such assistance immediately begins to build trust and helps overcome the awkwardness of trying to communicate across different cultural backgrounds. The particular help need not be related to the formal program objectives. It might range from directing someone to a relocated food stamp office to helping another to be reinstated on welfare, or to solve a credit problem. The point is simply to establish trust by rendering service.

This type of individual service, when given in the particular area of the health program, helps prove the value of the program to others. At this point it becomes easier to show how many more of these individual health problems can be solved by group or community action, and how health services can be made relevant to consumers.

A number of the programs studied in the Project dealt successfully with non-health matters. Here are some of the techniques used in several of them:

- Adult participation at group meetings increased when provision was made for a children's program at the same time. The kids enjoyed their activity and put pressure on their parents to come.

- In one community, existing outreach networks (Extension service, Y's, churches, etc.) were combined with the health care delivery system, and a coordinator and indigenous workers were employed to expand these relationships in program development.

- One group felt that transportation and babysitting expenses of low-income participants should be provided. If people missed work, their lost wages were compensated.

- The outreach workers developed their own strategies for recruitment based on their prior experience in their particular neighborhoods.

- Gathering household data for research purposes proved an effective recruitment tool to increase consumer use of health services. It gave the staff a better understanding of a community. This was reported by two large projects.

24

Summary

The anecdotal material collected demonstrates that the basis for initiating a health program or a new health service rarely begins with the rational approach of involving members of the consumer group in the identification of the need for the program. The initiation seems to rest with the concerned professional or someone with power. However, the success of the program was shown to be closely related to the extent of the involvement of those who would be affected.

The amount of time that was usually allowed to involve individuals and affect their behavior proved far too short. This lack of time was particularly significant in the preplanning stage. The difficulty of obtaining reliable information about consumers and their behavior was cited frequently.

An interpretation of health problems and services in a narrow manner was cited by practitioners as a very short-sighted approach. They suggested that time can be saved in the long run if one approaches consumer problems with a broader perspective.

References

1. Paul, Benjamin D. (ed.). Health, Culture and Community. Russell Sage Foundation, New York, 1955.
2. Ginzberg, Eli. Some Lessons of the 1960's, in The Great Society: Lessons for the Future; The Public Interest, No. 34, Winter, 1974.

III. Participation and Involvement —Crucial Ingredients

This section deals with the building of more effective health programs by encouraging the consumer's participation, and with the question of how best to create this partnership with the people staffing, administering and funding the program.

Distinctions Between Participation and Involvement

The concept of participation has been frequently used in the organization requirements of Federally funded health programs. Participation means taking part in some particular organizational arrangement. Involvement is participation carried a step further, to include understanding and personal commitment. Changes in the health care system can be brought about through participation, but changes in an individual's health behavior are brought about through his or her personal involvement.

Government legislation has created pressure to insure consumer participation. This legislation even goes so far as to state the percentage and kinds of consumers who should be represented on administrative and advisory boards. Such regulations may be useful in obtaining consumer viewpoints, but do not necessarily develop involvement.

Involvement can develop from active participation. It is sometimes thought of as the result of a fortunate coincidence—desirable but hard to create. But a consumer group can become involved when the members are provided with opportunities to learn about the problem. They need to gather information about possible solutions, to express their thoughts freely, and to have an equal voice in deciding what action should be taken. Often the consumers can be helped to assume responsible roles through a planned series of learning situations, in which each person is provided with the information that enables him or her to understand and choose among the various options.

Involvement is based on a recognition that individuals have a right to determine their own destiny and hence must be included in any decision which affects them individually, as a family, and as a community. When individuals are involved in this manner, the result can be predicted and identified.

In the programs studied by the Project it was found that the more consumers were involved in meaningful decisions, the greater was the achievement of the project's goals and the longer lasting the results. It was found that the only way to have true consumer involvement was to allow them to participate fully in the decision-making from the start.

Educational Basis for Involvement

Both basic and applied research in the field of education contain many excellent references which deal extensively with the "learning by doing" theory. This relates closely to the question of consumer participation in decisions. Rather than providing detailed information here, the reader is invited to use the bibliography for an expanded description of the methodology involved.

One caution which was given over and over by participants in the Project was that it was important to avoid only token consumer participation. Whether tokenism comes from a philosophic outlook, or simply an attitude, it is very quickly perceived by its victims. There is an understandable temptation to limit the participation and involvement of the consumer group, since it requires giving up a degree of control, with all the risks that people feel in such a situation. But when such fears can be overcome and a viewpoint arrived at, the program is ready to move forward. Quotations from two of the projects amplify the point:

- "It seems to take professionals six weeks to stop fearing consumers and another six weeks for consumers to stop being afraid of professionals."

- "We involved a number of the target population as soon as our grant was approved. To our surprise, since the community people had not been involved in the writing of the grant proposal, they perceived us as wanting to do something to them, make money on them, without caring about them or their real problems. Over time the staff learned that trust was a question which had to be settled in each training situation. To deal with trust, the Center staff had to first divest itself of power ... create for the trainees the freedom to make mistakes ... promote and even create an atmosphere in which self-determination becomes a reality. New options and alternatives, new possibilities to choose from, must be introduced where they are called for by the people involved."

An example of very extensive involvement of all groups concerned with the development of a program was described by a well-established agency. When Community Health Planning and Regional Medical Program funds became available to undertake a new approach to an old problem, the agency set up a series of actions which built a strong support base in the following manner:

The development of a community-wide health service delivery system for a low-income population of 30,000 in a county was planned and put into operation on a $40,000 budget for each health care referral center. There were the following kinds of participation at the beginning of the effort:

1. Twenty-five bi-lingual volunteers were immediately recruited to conduct the household consumer health survey in low-income neighborhoods and camps. The survey (362 families) was directed toward the determination of the impact the present health "system" was making on the lives of persons in these locations, toward uncovering additional health care needs and toward identifying grass-roots leadership.

2. Personal interviews were held with all (51) health providers to identify the extent to which the "system" was reaching out to the low-income population.

3. Health forums were held in nine communities with hundreds of health consumers and providers who represented all population groups. The participants were organized into small groups to consider the most important health needs in their communities and to discuss what resources were available.

4. An advisory committee for the program of the new health delivery system was organized with local health providers, consumers, and representatives from social services agencies.

5. Local neighborhood leadership was identified, recruited and trained to serve as Community Health Volunteers. The 45 "Block Leaders" were given three half-days of intensive training. These workers are paid a very small expense stipend per month. Each is identified by a name tag and a sign in a window of his or her home.

6. Working relationships were developed with existing social service centers and arrangements were made to train 22 members of their staffs in order to prepare them to serve the community as "health agents," or outreach workers.

Within a nine-month period, a Health Care Referral Center was established with a triage nurse, one full and one part-time Coordinator of Volunteers and a receptionist. In the first seven months of operation the Center handled 553 referrals, provided 1,342 manhours of training, and gave health education information to 3,930 families.

In addition to the core operation of the project, other activities were implemented. A "discharged patient" program was started to determine how the outreach networks could follow up on the needs of patients being discharged from hospitals. Several informal educational sessions were conducted during lunch hours and coffee breaks in the factories and packing houses within the target area. Cooperation was obtained with the State Dept. of Education project to provide the people in the area with the use of a mini-bus three full days per week to transport patients from the Center to the hospital.

Two thousand consumers have received assistance in the procurement of needed health care. Attendance at the Annual Pap Smear Clinic has tripled. Private health providers have accepted more low-income patients on the basis of state payment. The non-English-speaking consumer has increasingly accepted public health services. A six-month follow-up home evaluation is done on every patient who has been assisted by the Health Care Referral Center, and active participation of local people has continued to increase.

Monitoring Involvement

Many social forces have converged to bring about the requirement for consumer representation on boards and advisory committees. Yet those who are part of the group providing the services—usually members of the dominant community—express great concern over how these consumer representatives are to be selected, how long they should be retained, what functions they should perform, the conflicts that occur, and the benefits that are to be gained.

Recently, professional health and behavioral science journals have carried numerous articles analyzing the difficulties consumers have in participating on boards and committees with health professionals and other well-established members of the dominant community.

Project workshop participants cited a number of reasons why low-income consumers do not participate on boards and committees: inability to follow the professionals' technical language; different cultural patterns which determine how one participates in meetings; inconvenient meeting times and strange buildings; having their comments ignored; the use of Roberts Rules of Order; fear of some governmental authority holding their comments against them in another relationship (e.g., as a patient, welfare recipient, etc).

To overcome such fears providers need to:

1. Determine the physical location and circumstances that are most comfortable for the particular consumer group—e.g., large or small meetings, with or without children present, day or evening, etc., then accommodate to them.

2. Take a personal approach that is not threatening, even in subtle ways. Simple, non-technical language is certainly important, but if it is expressed in a patronizing way, it will only increase the social distance and alienate the consumer. Equally important is patient consideration and understanding of the ideas and sentiments of members of the consumer group.

3. Provide some tangible benefits as soon as possible, even if they involve being helpful to individuals in ways not directly related to the goals of the program.

Many different patterns of provider-consumer relationships were described. These ranged from open confrontation or rejection to mutual respect, trust and productive support. The following comments suggest what helped and what hindered the attainment of desirable relationships.

> ● "Although the directors of the agencies were brought in at the beginning of the planning, we found we had to backtrack to include staff before the program could be implemented."

• " 'Hard-to-reach' may characterize the provider segment more appropriately than the disadvantaged clientele."

• "In getting the program underway the health staff and the local leadership were not adequately educated with regard to the program objectives, so some locations used the outreach workers as 'technical assistants' rather than as community representatives helping the local leadership develop their own program under their own control, to identify community health problems and to find ways to better utilize health resources."

• "To obtain effective consumer participation, not only must the consumer develop knowledge and skills, but equally important, the professional, the providers and the dominant community must recognize the importance of the expertise and skills which the consumer can bring to the planning process."

• "The providers, too, must acquire special skills—the ability to listen; to communicate in simple terms . . . not to rely on technical terms or assume prior knowledge on the part of their audience. . . . It *is* possible to talk in simple terms without talking down to an audience; to accept the fact that low-income consumers are busy people, too; you need a readiness to give consumers credit for actions and insights and knowledge of consumers, cultural traditions, life styles and problems. . . ."

• "Community development does not produce 'instant consumers.' It provides for a development and educational process by which consumers acquire the skills, self-confidence, and community strength to contribute their own experience as consumers to such boards."

Flexibility in program design is essential. When the outreach workers and consumer participants begin to share with the staff "how it really is", the objectives, procedures and outcomes to be measured are perceived differently and must be adapted in order for the program to be relevant.

Ranking Participation

A scale was used during the Project to rank degrees of participation and involvement of four categories of participants—consumers, providers, administrators and policy makers. A bar chart showing how the programs ranked the degree of involvement of each category is presented on page 50.

An examination of the chart shows that the staff person interested in the educational aspects of a program most often goes about the preplanning and planning steps alone, that the administrator is brought into the planning more frequently than the consumer. In some situations the administrators are policy makers, so there is some redundancy in the data between these two categories.

The most revealing aspect of the chart is the limited amount of involvement by any category of participant in evaluation. The middle rating of "some involvement" usually was described as an

Involvement of Funders, Administrators, Providers, Consumers

In Four Phases of Programming Reported by 17 Programs

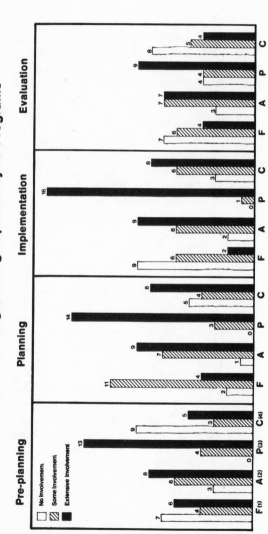

(1) Funders: Persons responsible for providing funds and setting criteria for these expenditures.

(2) Administrators: Decision-makers in the operating agency who allocate resources and determine overall policy direction.

(3) Providers: Staff members of the agency who provide services.

(4) Consumers: Members of the population who are expected to benefit from the program and/or use the services.

Specifics of involvement in the four phases of programming include:

1. Pre-planning: involvement in formulation of proposal, including definition of needs and resources, analysis of problem.

2. Planning: determination of goals, specific objectives, selection of method to achieve objectives and to measure outcomes.

3. Implementation: adaptation of activities and procedures on basis of staff and resources, provision of services and modification of services when needed.

4. Evaluation: determination of extent objectives were achieved; accountability of expenditures; interpretation of outcomes to others.

information-receiving rather than an action role in decision-making.

The 17 projects studied in depth revealed minimal involvement by consumers and funders during Stage I (Preplanning) and in Stage IV (Evaluation).

Getting Consumers Involved

One of the programs studied in the Project reported considerable success with involvement of consumers from the very outset in the preplanning stage. Here's how it came about:

A university staff had the good fortune of having had previous involvement with the community to be assisted. Building on this relationship, they did involve members of this target population in the preplanning stage. The staff met with representatives of consumer groups over a three-month period prior to preparation of the grant application and found they had a good grasp of the issues and problems. Their insights became essential to the planning for education of consumers in their role on health-related boards and committees.

This consumer group designated in the proposal that a consumer education committee be formed to guide the development of the training activities. The committee held a community meeting. Through the use of brain-storming groups, they defined and described the topics for the health training sessions to be held. They also decided on the scheduling of classes, became the admissions committee to check applications, chose a coordinator for each topic area, and developed an evaluation of the courses.

The community participants in the courses later requested more advanced courses in health and the health care system. Ten of the participants were selected to serve on a 23-member consumer/provider comprehensive health planning steering committee. Many others now are serving on patient councils or advisory boards for local hospitals and health agencies.

By giving priority to participation and involvement, the desires of the participants were included, and the resulting action developed strong support, making for a more effective program.

Summary

Participation and involvement help to insure the success of an educational program. Most people want to control their own destinies, and in a democratic society such as ours this is an accepted way of working. Learning is a process of choosing on the basis of experience from a variety of possible actions. Through the learning process, attitudes and values are formed which shape what individuals strive for and believe in. Through this process motivation is provided because the aspirations and goals are those of the participants.

The professional asks, "How do we adapt program ideas and services to the concerns, interests, ways of doing things, vocabulary, values and customs of our consumers? The easiest and most efficient way is to involve the people themselves in providing the guides and pathways for doing this. Among those to be involved are: Leaders within the target population; shopowners; clergy; newspaper, television and radio commentators who serve the target population; resident workers; and neighborhood groups.

Program planning and implementation must include all persons who are responsible for carrying out any part of the program: the consumer who will benefit, other persons who influence the individual's behavior, the health agency's governing body, administrators, staff at all levels, and persons associated with other agencies and institutions who can affect the outcomes of the program.

IV. Developing a Program

The most effective programs, especially among those directed toward minority or disadvantaged groups, utilized sound educational approaches which enabled consumers and providers to work together in program development. These included involving members of the target population in a variety of roles; developing working relationships with community leaders; and identifying needs, resources and community response patterns.

Gaining Entry to the Community

How does one gain entry into the minority setting? The most common approach is to select a member of the minority group who, often in the role of health aide or community leader, will solicit interest and cooperation and will try to motivate other members of his own group. Two of the oldest programs using minority members as community health aides are the Indian Health Service and the Alaska Native Health Service, but many more programs today employ this method of gaining entry. Two observations from other projects may offer guidance for those who wish to consider such an approach:

- "The strength of the program depends

upon the kind of training and supervision the outreach worker has. The worker must have organizational skills, be able to put program components into logical sequence, define problems, identify resources, and develop programs. The individual also must be sensitive to the life situation of people and aware of techniques of helping them to make effective use of their own strengths to help themselves."

• "Each aide functions differently and must be permitted to work in his/her own way. The agency should only set parameters and provide professional back-up for its work. The aide will uncover things we never thought of as important. Then we must realign our objectives."

Community workers are subject to many pressures. They, too, need recognition. They may have a personal agenda that transcends their service motivation. Often they have personal needs which are met by solving the personal needs of others. They are torn between the desire to achieve quick results and the longer process of letting the community develop its own leadership, make its own mistakes, and learn through the process. They must learn there is a time to act and a time to wait, with emphasis heavily on the waiting, the listening, the suggesting, and querying. The age of the worker is not important. Maturity is.

Here are observations made during the workshops on ways to recruit outreach workers and to improve communication between them and the health professionals:

• "The selection of outreach workers was

a combination of individual interviews and a group/workshop interview. In the group interview applicants could be observed in their relationships with peers when discussing community problems and how they would deal with them.''

● ''You need a 'bridging' person to take ideas from the outreach workers to the professionals and administrators in the system. Good suggestions surface among employees, but everyone is afraid to express an idea or act on it for fear of losing his job.''

● ''Center staff provided expertise in their respective service areas and assisted in staff development of the outreach worker. The staff served as resource persons during training, which made communication and coordination of services easier.''

Using members of the minority group to gain entry and acceptance is not a guarantee of success. Some cautions were expressed by members of the project staffs:

● ''My black face isn't enough to get me accepted in a Black community; I must join them in all their activities. They may treat me one way on a one-to-one basis, and entirely differently in a group meeting.''

● ''It is crucial that the staff person be known in the community as someone who is sensitive to people's problems. If a committee member loses a job or there's a death in the family, you should wait. It's wrong to go ahead without every individual.''

• ''There are many people who care, who cry a lot, but who can't do anything. We in the Valley judge people by what they do. If they sit in the office and rip off a salary, we don't accept them. But we'll accept an Anglo from New York if he works.''

• ''In a polarized community, local staff can be disastrous. By appointing a community resident to staff, the outside agency is in effect designating a community leader, preempting the community's responsibility.''

Patterns of Provider-Consumer Relationships

People who have always lived in one place come to accept things the way they are—to seem almost unaware of the possibilities for change and improvement. It helps to find marginal people who run into problems and seek outside solutions; they are better able and more willing to explain the problems and health beliefs of the group to you. The employment and training of outreach workers is not limited to belonging to just one group or the other. Their new position also gives them power to do something about the problems.

The relationships between people providing health care and those receiving it ranged from open confrontation or rejection to mutual respect, trust, and productive support. Minority or low-income consumers exhibit different patterns of behavior, which often create apprehension and confusion among professionals. Here are some examples:

- During the training sessions for inner-city Black outreach workers, the staff observed the following pattern of interaction: There was, at virtually all times, an apparently harsh, critical impatience among the trainees toward one another. Loud talk and anger were heatedly expressed. However, the tirades were generally followed with laughter and joking and an apparent feeling of good will. Staff discovered that this highly emotional group style was a reflection of a cultural life style; it was simply different.

- "The group sometimes has to attack you as a representative of the 'system' in order to gain solidarity . . . but then they're willing to work with you to solve problems."

- "Some consumer leaders come to meetings with their constituencies. They have to perform for them during the meeting, but are willing to negotiate with you at another time on a one-to-one basis."

- "To gain the confidence of immigrants you must remove the fear of being deported. They need someone who is a member of their culture, who lives there and can be visible; they need a person who is bilingual and can help them with their pressing problems—employment, housing, money."

The myth that the poor seldom volunteer was found untenable by workshop participants. They commented further that getting people involved as volunteers brought a lot of returns besides the savings in dollars and cents, or reaching the particular objective of the program. The volunteers themselves became fulfilled; they felt important again.

As the results with volunteers show, a provider-consumer relationship may not turn out as expected, or even as happened in the past. It was found best to be open-minded when introducing changes, rather than to assume that a response will be of one particular kind or another. Everyone gains confidence in a problem-solving approach that requires mutual cooperation and assumes that part of the answer lies on each side.

Community Leadership and Power Structure

Several patterns of community leadership, power structure, and the influence of past history were brought out in the Project. These patterns are important because they affect the acceptance of outsiders and the changes in the health system they are promoting.

One of the findings of the Project was that the community was often fragmented, with an entrenched leadership or self-appointed leaders. In such a situation it is difficult to involve the rest of the community in assuming responsibility and making decisions. By rotating the leadership of the group in the early stages of a program, it was found that power could be diffused and the basis for decisions broadened to involve others.

When a leader is chosen to preside for a whole

year, attention is most often focused on the person rather than the issue. Therefore, it needs to be clarified and accepted that the role of the leader is not to express views, but only to keep order and to make sure everyone gets a chance to speak. It is necessary to insure that every member of a group has an opportunity to develop participation and leadership skills. One observation made was that excessive competition for the chairmanship might be cooled by pointing out its obligations and disadvantages. Rotating the responsibilities not only allows each person to develop new skills, but also to develop a better self-image.

Development of task-oriented groups is another way to sidestep entrenched leadership. Task forces or ad hoc groups develop confidence, specialized expertise and factual knowledge. They broaden leadership potential and give every member the opportunity to express his or her needs. They improve channels of communication with groups and resources outside the community.

Being responsible to a constituency that is informed is vital. In one community consumers used the elective process to change their representative, who they felt was not representing their interests in dealing with the dominant community. In another situation persistent questioning by others in a group forced the representative to share information. In a third project area, a policy was made to have two or three consumers participate in any meeting or consultation to keep the representatives "honest."

If one attempts to select city-wide leaders rather than having the population of the community involved select and develop its own leaders, then community education comes from the top down, rather than being developmental. In such a case the majority of the low-income consumers remain followers rather than participants or initiators. Consequently fewer people become personally involved and actively committed to the program, and its effectiveness is reduced.

Flexibility in program design is necessary if a strong community group is to emerge. Certain dynamics are at work. There are times when a community is ready to respond and times when it is not. Internal politics, conditions and moods play an important part and cannot be ignored. Development cannot be forced.

Variations in patterns of holding meetings were described by participants in the workshops. Staff working in communities of newly arrived Asians noted that an idea or program had to be aired first in a large community meeting so everyone could recognize that it had general acceptance. Only then could the staff move to small neighborhood groups to develop specific plans.

In contrast, Alaskan natives do not respond in village-wide meetings, but will raise their questions and participate in discussions when the meetings are in homes or other places where they feel at ease.

Consumer participation in meetings with providers, face-to-face discussions and confrontations with providers, and consumer involvement in the development of joint planning efforts and problem-solving sessions can break down the mystique surrounding physicians and demystify the whole area of health care.

Staff can produce an information sheet which provides community people with the basic information they need to participate effectively in discussions and meetings with the providers and professionals. This has the further advantage of preventing any one segment of the community from monopolizing information for its own use and advantage.

One of the difficulties that may be encountered is a polarized community. Whether the polarization has occurred around an issue or around the leadership does not matter. The problem is that any public forum can be used to disrupt programs and create open confrontation; hence one may need to have small neighborhood meetings and involve consumers in problem-solving task forces, rather than holding public meetings.

Past history of community decision-making may be an asset or a deterrent in planning health care projects. It is quite possible that a community may have been embroiled in a controversy over one part of a program, which then stalls the entire effort. One of the most traumatic subjects can be the location of a new hospital or clinic. Arguments about the location can delay or block provision of the service for an indefinite time. Getting agreement on smaller, less controversial subjects at first may make it easier to cut through any bad feelings.

If a group is organized around a single purpose, once that goal has been achieved, its members seem to need a period of rest before they are ready to attack a new problem. Maintaining cohesiveness and unity of a group which has come together around a basic concern, particularly if controversy is high, is an important internal goal. Small successes that are visible and concrete are essential.

These experiences illustrate the importance of community organization. A careful analysis of the forces at work in a community is essential before deciding how and when to proceed with problem-solving strategies.

Using Outside Assistance

Among the projects studied, assistance was frequently used from state, regional or national sources, or outside consultants, when information was not available locally. There were beneficial results when adequate preparation was made in advance.

Travel to another community or site by a local group interested in developing health education programs also proved beneficial, although it was not as common. The opportunity to observe in person how other people have struggled to produce a health service or program helps develop a sense of balance in one's own situation.

Health professionals should be encouraged to call on outside consultants. Not only can they obtain technical data and other useful information, but they can also learn how to help local groups become more familiar with the accepted ways of conducting business and arriving at decisions. Such outside contacts, whether through visits or use of a consultant, can help staff members in unforeseen ways. For instance, it is easy to take for granted that disadvantaged or minority groups can accept middle-class ways of conducting meetings, reaching decisions, using data, and other standard procedures. Unfortunately, the social distance is not always apparent. Unfamiliarity with common means of communication such as the telephone may appear incredible to the middle-class professional, but learning how to use such devices and feeling comfortable in doing so may be one of the first educational experiences needed.

Gathering Data

Descriptive or "soft" data are often more useful in the health education program, than are the
usual statistical data required in research work. In
all but one of the projects studied at the workshops,
data were used for program guidance and monitor-
ing instead of research for comparative purposes.

Important questions for data collection are:

• To whom is the program directed?

• What are the goals of the program?

• What information is available about the
population which will suggest how they
might be expected to respond?

• What is the present situation?

• What resources are available?

• What is the desired outcome?

The answers to these questions are the basis for
sound program development. However, seldom
were all of these questions posed, nor were the
implications of the information gathered fully utilized.

In the projects reviewed, a number of data
gathering techniques were used. Sources of data for
the health education program are both objective
and subjective. Objective data from hospitals and
social agencies may be available in surveys made
for other purposes. Census tract information and
National Health Survey reports also may provide
important insights. For instance, the National

Health Survey, which reports on illness problems of low-income people, has been used productively in conjunction with the findings of a local survey.

An extensive example is cited to illustrate how a new alliance was formed to gather data and analyze a problem. The approach was to involve those who provide service with those who use the service in order to gain each other's perspectives on the problem and solutions. Hence improvement of a clinic system was the focus of one project by a group of staff-level providers, consumers, and representatives of community agencies, who became concerned with the poor quality of care being provided. Data become more relevant and action more likely if those who make changes are involved in data collection and analysis of the data gathered. The data gathered resulted in the decision to do the following:

1. Establish a screening system by which missing charts and requested laboratory work might be found the day prior to a patient's appointment.

2. Determine a realistic ceiling for the number of patients to be seen.

3. Develop routines to assure that appropriate workups were done on all patients.

4. Establish clear patient counseling and specific follow-up responsibilities of staff.

5. Devise patient information cards to keep track of vital demographic, social and medical information.

6. Reorganize routines for doing laboratory work so the results would be consistently obtained.

7. Clarify procedures on prescription writing and handling walk-in patients.

In the past the clerical and nursing staff did not have consistent assignments or clear responsibilities. This led to much clerical work that was unnecessary or was being done by professional staff. The waste and confusion was frustrating to the doctors, nurses and receptionists. The toll it took on patients included exceedingly long clinic visits, countless unnecessary reordered tests, and unnecessary return visits to the clinic.

When an integrated service approach was tried, it had the following effect on patient care:

1. The "kept appointment rate" improved from 53 percent to 71 percent in one year through institution of a staggered appointment system to replace the block appointment system.

2. Patients now call more consistently when they need to cancel appointments.

3. There has been a noticeable change in patient-staff relations. Patients take more affirmative roles in their health care by inquiring about their medication and method of treatment, and in their concern about wanting to be seen by "their doctor."

4. The follow-up letters and telephone calls made on every missed appointment have encouraged patients to obtain and keep new appointments.

5. These improvements helped the clinic in two ways: The cost of duplicating "lost" tests was eliminated, and tests performed were charged for. Previously only 58 percent of the completed laboratory work reached the patient's chart. Over a six-month period, 59 missing laboratory results were recovered; this saved $885 through the collection of laboratory fees for services rendered. Many staff hours were saved on blood work alone, which saved $1000 to $2000 in a year.

The household interview was one of the most frequently used techniques of data collection in the projects studied. Not only did it supply the data requested, but it also served as a recruiting device for obtaining program participants. However, several project participants warned that low-income consumers are tired of being surveyed by "outsiders," particularly when the surveyor tends to profit financially or professionally.

One project described the variety of functions which can be served by survey methods:

> • "A consumer household survey was conducted in the low-income neighborhood and migrant camps in order to determine the impact of the health system on people's lives, to uncover additional unmet needs, and to identify grass roots leadership. All health providers were also surveyed to identify the extent to which the system was reaching out to the low-income people. Goals of the project were based on these findings."

Interviews with key individuals from the group being served and with staff members in touch with the community can shed light on the nature of a community's problems and attitudes.

This subjective information can be quantified and compared with similar information from other communities with beneficial results. One project staff member said, "As a matter of fact, subjective data and evaluation are impressive. Everyone knows how bad that hospital is; they know about that one case where someone had this terrible experience and, Lord knows, it travels like wildfire." The situation can be related to observations that there may be many more instances just like it. Then attention can be directed to this finding and solutions sought.

Learning something about the local situation can be important in ways that are hard to foresee when gathering information. For instance:

- If young people are not keeping their clinic appointments, it may be simply that they have been scheduled for times when they are supposed to be in school.

- It would be a mistake to plan meetings at night in a high-crime area.

- It may be an advantage to provide pencil, paper and a brochure in an area in which illiteracy is common and reading is a prized skill.

When time and resources were invested at the outset in learning about a community, ethnic group or an institution in terms of their patterns of communication, influence, decision-making and power, realistic and acceptable program plans emerged. Initial contacts may not yield all the information desired, nor is it likely that the situation will remain static. It is therefore necessary to engage in continual fact-finding and reappraisal of the expectations, barriers and actions which occur. To mobilize community resources effectively to solve a problem and gain support for a new program, the staff must be able to adapt its services and actions to the various forces at work.

In this section observations about steps in developing a program were provided. Cautions and suggestions were cited with regard to (1) gaining entry into a community; (2) anticipating the response of the population; (3) locating and using outside resources and (4) data gathering techniques.

V. Implementing a Program

The implementation stage must be planned to include all persons who are responsible for carrying out any part of the program. This includes the consumer who will benefit, other persons who influence their behavior, the health agency's governing body, the administrator's staff at all levels, and persons associated with other agencies and institutions who can affect the outcomes of programs.

The formulation of a plan of operation may have been well thought out in the planning phase[1]; however, the details of what, when, where and how a program will operate often reveal a number of unrealistic expectations. These may be based on inadequate information or may stem from changes which occurred between the time the initial plan was designed and when it was implemented.

A frequently referred-to program scheme calls for looking at the problem cause, contributing factors, barriers to change and consideration of alternative ways of resolving the problem before instituting a program. Among the programs reviewed, there was little evidence in the documentation that formal consideration had been given to these issues, especially to the procedure of reviewing possible alternative solutions. A look at the approach taken in the examples cited suggests, however, that intuitively the cause and contributing factors may have indeed been examined:

- "A referral system throughout the health institutions was created. All disciplines were active and introduced patients, their siblings, and other community members to project-sponsored activities."

- "Although the directors of the agencies were brought in at the beginning of the planning, we found we had to backtrack to include staff before the program could be implemented."

- "To obtain effective consumer participation, not only must the consumer develop his knowledge and skills, but equally important, the professional providers and members of the dominant community must recognize the importance of the expertise and skills which the consumer can bring to the planning process."

- "An educational approach can help all concerned to understand and respect the differing contributions, functions, roles and competencies of the professional and the consumer."

- "Center staff provided expertise in their respective service areas and assisted in staff development of the outreach workers. The staff's participation as resource persons during training also facilitated communication and coordination of services."

Staff Considerations

Preparation of the staff to understand the application of certain educational principles, to anticipate some barriers and constraints, and to be prepared to try different educational approaches and methods with the consumers can save embarrassment and inconsistencies in working with them.

As services are extended or expanded to low-income and minority groups, the existing staff needs an opportunity to explore alternative solutions to the problems which arise. They need to be able to consider a variety of strategies so they can choose one or a combination which will best meet the situation.

Health workers are best prepared to undertake new programs with consumers by working in collaboration with other members of the organization. The process requires continual examination of how the actions undertaken are working out and what can be done to facilitate improvement. This approach differs from an in-service training where one schedules learning experiences focused on improving skills and knowledge. The changes which are made depend upon the way the staff analyzes and diagnoses what is happening in their operation. In order for this process to succeed, an organizational climate is required in which the staff has the freedom as well as the responsibility to develop more effective practices.

All members of the staff who will be associated with the program need to have an opportunity to examine and discuss their responsibilities and functions and how they relate to one another. They should be involved as a staff group in determining procedures, developing and pretesting record-keeping forms, identifying referral sources, and establishing outreach plans to bring services to members of the target group, on the basis of the priorities dictated by the objectives. The staff group should create feedback mechanisms to obtain prompt and complete information on how the plan is working, how the staff is functioning and how well communications are being maintained within and between cooperating agencies and groups.

- "The employment of outreach workers who were members of the population to be served proved to be an effective means of reaching individuals and groups within their framework of understanding and action. Success with the addition of this type of staff was dependent upon the integration of the new worker into the overall staff effort and included technical supervision both in terms of health facts and educational methodology."

Changing Direction

It is often necessary to define the program broadly enough to meet changing emphases, but it is also necessary to be concrete so that objectives can be measured. This requires creativity in meeting new situations that are still within the broad purpose of the program. Here is how others have expressed this need for adaptability:

- "If staff are hired to implement a plan developed by others, they tend to develop their own methods and goals. It is extremely important they be involved in the development of the proposal. If not, it is essential that at the outset enough time be devoted to orientation and discussion of the philosophy, aims and methods.''

● ''There is no prototype or model that can be picked up whole and used in other communities, and any proposed procedure must be flexible and subject to adaptation. No two communities are at the same level of organization or sophistication. No two communities have the same resources or identical problems. No two communities stand in the same relation to the rest of their city or area.''

● ''Administrators must recognize that policies, plans, and programs addressed to human behavior require more precise information and understanding of complex social processes. They need to strike a workable balance between rigorous design and methods with the situational realities in which the program functions.''

The situation remains fluid, even after the project gets underway, because new information generated by the program itself may bring about a shift in objectives. One program director pointed to the need to ''stop a minute along the way and re-examine objectives.''

Another project staff member said, ''Working in a living community is a very complex thing—you take a string and see where it leads.'' As goals are changed there may be a problem in how to interpret the new goals and changes to administrators and funders. Will they be able to go along? Often there needs to be a compromise between community goals and agency goals. Here is how others have urged a sort of "structured flexibility."

- "Pretests yield objective data which help to indicate whether or not specific steps in program planning development are being successfully carried out, but they do not obtain evidence of program effectiveness. ... During developmental stages of a program there is a need to identify barriers to success at a time when changes can be made easily and at a minimum cost."

- "Our health education program is simple in its conception. We see a problem in the clinic and we tackle it step by step. We ask what we can do and start somewhere, no matter how trivial the beginning seems. We are open to dealing with any issue, no matter how small, that stands in the way of our goal, which is simply the delivery of quality health care. The process of change is a lot more complicated than the goal. The task is neither overwhelming nor impossible. The essence for workable change seems to be simplicity and a clear understanding of goals."

In all of the interchange of views and experiences in the Project, change was shown to be an unsettling experience for everyone—especially when it is someone else bringing about a change that affects you. The concerns consumers expressed about being involved in determining what changes need to be made, by whom and when and how, were voiced equally by the administrators and health workers.

Examples of Educational Methods

Throughout the previous sections various educational methods were described as part of how one gains entry into a community, gathers data, obtains involvement and develops programs. In this section specific educational methods have been singled out to illustrate the various ways one specifically plans educational experience for consumers, staff, administrators and all others involved in the program.

The examples illustrate a variety of approaches: the individual approach, small group discussions and outreach to community groups. However, since many educational plans involve more than one method, the material cannot be presented in distinct categories. Subtitles have been used to stress the unique thrust of the examples cited.

Creating and Distributing the Message

The concept of involvement of consumers and providers in determining (1) what information is relevant to the population, (2) in what form it should be presented, and (3) how it can best be channeled to the group was used by a number of the programs.

Consumers and providers had a problem-solving experience working together to make videotapes and other educational materials directly related to the consumer problems being seen in a hospital outpatient department. The topics varied from how to use the clinic to lead poisoning, immunization, and the meaning of comprehensive health care. Members of the target population were attracted to the messages because they could identify with the content and pictures. The health staff were receptive to using the educational materials because they were relevant to their concerns. Both groups learned a great deal about each other's way of viewing the problems and potential solutions. Thus the process, as well as the product, provided education.

When a small group of Mexican-American women were brought together to develop a cancer education program for their population, they evolved an interesting approach. After reviewing existing publications they themselves decided what they wanted to learn, and in what order they wanted to learn it. They surveyed other women to find out what they wanted to know and how it should be presented. This resulted in a booklet, "Hablaremos Sobre Cancer Dentro de la Familia," which means "Let's Talk About Cancer Within the Family."

Distribution of these booklets was personalized through a "family plan," rather than relying on physical distribution to the neighborhood. This family plan consisted of the individual drawing a family tree which shows a rough listing of names and addresses of all family members that the individual can reach. The booklet is mailed or delivered in person and follow-up discussions are held. Then the new persons reached are encouraged to "round robin" the booklet to others. Each woman in the original group spread the message to as many as 20 others and sometimes to relatives in other states and Mexico.

In this experience members of the group become involved in developing their own material, and in the process provide the agency staff with an understanding of the communication channels and cultural patterns of the consumer group.

A worker from within the community to be served was commonly employed as a channel for transmitting educational messages. As staff of one of the neighborhood health centers put it, "We are committed to the realization that the most effective change agents are persons from the very populations with whom we work."

In the Vista Bi-Lingual Health Aides Project, a cooperative venture of several health and social welfare agencies in Hawaii, bi-lingual health aide volunteers carried on outreach programs. They also conducted area meetings quarterly between newly-arrived immigrants and persons giving health service to acquaint the newcomers with the workings of the American health system. Person-to-person discussions were supplemented by printed materials developed or translated into Philippino, Korean and Samoan.

To help overcome traditional distance between institution and community, the health education unit at Roosevelt Hospital took part in neighborhood festivals such as block parties and health fairs. A health game was created that proved entertaining to players and gave the game sponsor a chance both to deliver a painless health message and to build a greater rapport with potential and actual users of the clinic's services.

A health staff, in addition to developing special written materials to help explain clinic operations, enlisted the talents of a neighborhood artist who depicted and identified the functions of clinic staff. These pictures are displayed in the clinic to familiarize clients with people whom they will see.

The small-group discussion method was used extensively as learning experiences for consumers and staff. The focus varied from improving interrelationships among providers and consumers to problem solving and to more effective consumer participation on decision-making committees and boards.

Identifying and Solving Problems

A small-group discussion format also was used in a project where the goal was not to prescribe specific solutions to child-rearing problems, nor to designate what should be discussed, but rather to involve parents in discussion groups where they could find strength, motivation, information, and know-how for a fresh approach to problems and people. The discussion topics came out of the group. They were asked what they needed, what they felt, and what they wanted to do. The professionals presented the options. The parents made the choices. The group discussions elicited these responses:

1. They relaxed tensions and fears. "It was more than meetings. It was company . . . friends like I never had before. I could talk about problems and find someone who would understand. Just talking about problems gives you courage to do something about them."

2. They created self-confidence: "It helped me understand my children better by finding out that other parents had the same problem; we came to a solution."

3. They aroused a wish for change: "I can't go back to living the same way after this."

4. They brought new attitudes and expectations: "It gives me a new idea of myself and of the possibilities of the changes that can be made."

The decisions on what to do belonged to the participants. "They opened playgrounds, paved streets, battled tuberculosis, erected traffic signs, sent kids to camp, enforced housing codes, established surplus food distribution centers, got out the vote, and started adult education programs.''

Workshops

As inter-city community groups became interested in health affairs, some saw the need for training and sought the help of experts in university training programs and independent centers. Experienced staff members helped groups increase their knowledge of health matters and expand their abilities to manipulate and negotiate with the system through workshop sessions. The Texas Consumer Participation Project employed a wide range of methods to increase the skills of both low-income consumers and members of the "dominant" community. Visits to other cities and projects as well as participation in national conferences helped build the confidence of consumers. Joint participation of consumers and providers in workshops helped break down some barriers. Skillful staff members drew the attention of members of the dominant community to the difference between their ways of asserting power and pressure and the means available to low-income people.

Problem-solving workshops can be an effective technique for imparting information, but they require careful planning by consumers and staff. They should have a limited and specific focus. They must in truth be work sessions and provide for involvement of those attending. It takes time to be sure that all questions are raised and answered. Groups should be kept small (10 to 15 participants) with an informed resource person. Factual material should be prepared in advance so that attenders can have something concrete to take away with them. Low-income consumers need travel funds, free meals and occasionally stipends to cover costs of baby sitters or to compensate for job income loss.

Role Playing

Role playing can be effective, particularly when the role assigned offers the participants an opportunity to portray the way they perceive the behaviors of another person with whom they are expected to interact (e.g., a patient portraying a physician discussing a diagnosis with the patient). The use of this technique should be limited to a time when the participants have developed an open-end trusting relationship. The roles assigned and situation to be dramatized also must be carefully selected to avoid unsettling feelings about the intensity of the problem or deep concerns inappropriate for open discussion among members of the group.

Staff Meetings and Team Development

To deepen staff workers' appreciation of education for health, weekly health education project committee meetings were held at several projects. Present at one of these meetings were the director of the children's and youth service, the hospital administrative staff, and supervisory staff. Lectures, discussions, and involvement of staff in identification of problem areas and preparation of written materials were used to add to staff workers' understanding and to deepen their commitment to the project.

In Watts the providers and consumer representatives were brought together to work as a team. "The team developed programs to deal with a variety of community health problems. These problems included obesity, sickle-cell anemia, blood poisoning and hypertension.''

Around each topic the team works together to develop the following:

1. ways of ascertaining current knowledge and practices through various pre-tests;

2. introductory statements or overviews;

3. statistics to point out the extent of the problem;

4. a summary of medical aspects of the problem;

5. poems, songs, skits, short stories to dramatize the problem;

6. a fact sheet;

7. a short film strip or announcement to use on radio or television.

These ''productions'' are presented by team members to a variety of community groups such as parent-teacher associations, church groups, social clubs, tenants associations, youth groups, patients, and others. The team and its productions are flexible, utilizing a lot of audience participation and striving for relevance with each audience or target group. Perhaps the most noteworthy aspect of this approach is the fact that the preventive health team teaches its process to the organization it works with. This organization in turn can develop similar teams to present the topics to still other groups.

Preparation of Board Members

When community people are called on to participate on community boards, they must develop new knowledge and skills. The consumer training program of one Midwest community was assigned to be as much like the regular agency activities as possible so that, in addition to acquiring information and concepts, consumers could learn to use that information and those skills for effective participation. Autonomous action of board members was to be an expected outcome. Therefore, even though staff initiated the formation of the training group, they withdrew from leadership as soon as they had developed the members' leadership capacity. The group learned to develop an agenda, to understand the dynamics of interactions among participants, to test their roles as capable legitimate members, and to educate themselves on information and opinion needed for decisions on community health matters.

One-to-One Education

In many health problems it is essential to develop an individualized message which can help a person understand information requiring his action on a situation unique to him. Some examples of how education was individualized follow:

Often educational messages need to be introduced through stages which include the use of groups and one-to-one teams. A highly charged topic, family planning, was broached in one community clinic first in a group information-giving session with individual instruction and counseling coming only at a later session. This gave the participants an opportunity to mull over and discuss the questions before working on individual decisions.

Health centers providing direct health services most commonly conducted a generalized health information service along with the provision of care. Hence, each staff member providing service is expected to give individual counseling and instruction. In these settings the feasibility or opportunity for group or class instruction in consumer settings is not great. In-service training programs spent their resources and efforts on improving the human relations and communications skills of the direct providers.

The Problem-Oriented Medical Record is being used[2] as the basis for involving the patient in medical care. Only the patient can answer the following questions:

1. Is this an accurate description of me in my role and interactions in society?

2. Is the subjective data under each problem accurate?

3. Are the plans under each problem clearly understood by me?

Those involved in the use of the POMR state it is a "useful tool for the creation of a true partnership in health care between the physician and the patient. It also provides a valuable audit function. And 97 percent of the patients are reassured and motivated by reviewing their own health care data."

Consumers often lack the whole range of information and skills they need to cope with, not only health problems, but such problems as housing, employment, and education. The educational method used by Indiana's Forty Family Project was to link families in poverty with sponsors from middle-income groups who served as guides and models for improvement. Education was then provided to both families by nutrition and environmental health workers who learned that the educational message needed to include suggestions on how to carry out the actions they recommended. For example, recommending that a family preserve its garden produce also required instructing them on the proper utensils and methods to use. The follow-up utilizing the information became a joint project between the two matched families.

Using Community Networks

Getting specific information about health services and problems to all segments of a target population requires the use of many techniques. In each situation the communicator needs to locate the channels which are appropriate for the message and effective in reaching the individuals. The route is often not a direct one but rather through informal leaders, social groups, and many specifically created networks.

The old principle of "go where the people are" is applied in a Florida Model Cities Health Project. Much of this health education is carried out through community work by way of group presentations. The presentations may be carried out at youth halls, day care centers, Model Cities public health units, and at several atypical locations For example:

- "There are a great many barber shops and beauty salons in the Model City area and many people are reached at this time with little or no inconvenience to them. The female Health Education Assistants hold informal discussions with the patrons of the beauty salons about family health, and the male Health Education Assistants take a film and carry on informal discussions on health concerns with the patrons of the barber shops.

The consumer health education demonstration project—Program Outreach—in Baltimore used staff to reach into the neighborhoods to communicate with teenage groups on street corners, homes, and other popular gathering places. In tune with the project's commitment to consumer participation in decision-making, the staff involved 'teens and parents in planning and organizing them around wholesome, developmental activities in response to the adolescents' felt needs. As a comprehensive health education program the first eight months of Program Outreach involved over 3500 individuals, many (300) of whom functioned as adult and 'teen leaders on behalf of the Project.

Working With the School

The sickle cell anemia medical advisory committee of the Cleveland Academy of Medicine and the Cleveland Medical Association, in response to a request from the city's public schools for help in education about sickle cell anemia, developed a curriculum for use by the schools. The program was planned for Junior or Senior High School students, based on the premise that a teenager is "especially receptive to learning more about his body and health and may be unusually receptive to sickle cell education programs whose results may have personal relevance. He's also available for testing and counseling."

The program was built around the existing science curriculum. The first approach utilized outside Black medical experts and audio-visual materials, and provided question-and-answer sessions. The first attempt, however, proved unsatisfactory, since the teachers were not prepared to respond to the questions of the students once the experts had left.

A revised approach involved the science teacher directly in the program. Through his participation and in-service workshop sessions the teacher became an independent expert in the area. A student work booklet and leaders' guides for the teachers was produced. The curriculum used a film to demonstrate how the trait is identified in the laboratory. It also provided exercises to show the transmission of genetic traits, and it gave simulated real-life situations for discussion of ethical and social issues associated with sickle-cell anemia.

Summary

The numerous examples cited have demonstrated that there is no single, fool-proof recipe for the selection of the best educational method. The method must be suited to the particular consumer and the particular situation in order to encourage consumers to take desirable health actions consistent with their goals, values, and life styles.

Education is more likely to be relevant and effective when it is made part of a health program with defined actions and when it is adapted to identified subgroups within the population. The benefits from the educational process are often synergistic and not specific to a single educational effort. Education sometimes may result in immediate action with limited benefits. Often it produces delayed results that take as long as a generation to change patterns of behavior. Specific benefits are useful, but they are not final evidence of effectiveness.

The importance of enlisting the consumer in the program is cited by these statements of health workers:

● "When new steps are contemplated for the project, we actively enlist the support of the people in whose lives we anticipate intervening. The power of the project is its willingness to learn first and act later."

● "Three years of intensive work in two disparate communities have validated the assumption that consumers of health services . . . that is, the people who live where the problems are . . . can identify those problems, can organize to produce solutions to those problems, and can work with providers."

References

1. Paul C. Buchanan, "The Concept of Organization Development, or Self-Renewal, As a Form of Planned Change", in Concepts for Social Change, edited by Goodwin Watson, National Training Laboratories, 1967, Washington, D. C.
2. Bouchard, R. E., Eddy, W. M., Tufo, H. M., Twitchell, J. C., Van Buren, H. C. and Bedford, Louise. "The Patient and His P.O.M.R." *Quality Assurance of Medical Care*, Monograph, Feb., 1973, Regional Medical Program Service, Health Services, and Mental Health Administration, DHEW, Washington, D.C.

VI. Assessing Accomplishment

This section deals with the evaluation of health education programs—the appraisal of what happened and how effective it was in carrying out the purpose of the project.

This is the era of accountability and evaluation, with demands from all sides for some measurement of outcome of effort and cost. The projects studied reflected a variety of reasons for evaluation being undertaken, not unlike the ones reported in the literature by Arnold[1] and Greene.[2] The projects showed that evaluation was used both as a scientific tool and a political tool, with use of rational and scientific criteria as well as advocacy criteria.

Attitudes Toward Evaluation

The subject of program evaluation usually brought forth an emotional response. Attitudes ranged all the way from the negative "I evaluate only what the funders require" to the more positive view of wanting to know what really took place. Here are examples of the different views:

• "There's no program that shouldn't be evaluated. Time, money, people are precious; whenever money, time or people are spent, the outcome should be evaluated for the benefit of others and to learn yourself."

• "It's possible to measure the changes brought about through accumulating good baseline data before the program is set up. Gather the data, as tedious as this may be. Hire outside assistance and analyze data. Ask yourself, what are we doing, the results of which are measurable? Primary prevention through education won't be measurable on a short term basis; early intervention before conditions become serious, perhaps we can measure. But have we gathered the right data?"

• "I don't think evaluation per se has merit; there's no point in evaluating some programs. What's it for, how does it affect the future, and what's going to be done with it? These questions need to be asked about each evaluation."

• "How do you measure results when you're talking about social change and human involvement? It may be that five years from now one of the people who took part will assume a major community leadership role. Delayed results are hard to measure."

• "I really question whether evaluation

responses to funding sources are truly honest. It's human nature to set your best foot forward. You may have to go back to that source of funds again. You are not going to say, 'We messed that up.' "

It appeared that the projects which were able to carry out a reasonable degree of evaluation were ones where tracers and indicators were identified early in the planning stages and where mid-point benchmarks were specified in advance. In projects where skepticism and lack of confidence prevailed, the evaluation required more time and greater staff attention.

Limitations of Numbers

No discussion of evaluation would be complete without reference to the "numbers game"—the frustrating but usually necessary attempt to express a series of complicated behavior changes in numbers alone. It is to the credit of the directors of our 17 projects that they provided a frank and open look at how objectives were set and outcomes measured. As described by one project:

● "Administrators are forced to indicate how many pamphlets were distributed, how many referrals were made, how many people attended a film showing. Program administrators are seldom asked questions such as the following: Did the family change its behavior patterns? Do its members understand the value of immunizations? Did Mrs. A. have a Pap smear? Did Mr. B. clean up the potential rats' nest in his backyard? Did the city tear down the

unsanitary and unsightly house? Did the
health department change the hours of the
neighborhood clinic? The numbers in answer to these questions may be small but
very meaningful."

Numbers can describe access to people and
exposure to certain kinds of messages. But along
with the numbers, individual episodes of help or
case histories of problem-solving should be sought.
These illuminate the nature and intensity of need,
as well as provide the evaluator with a better feel
for the situation in those programs where numbers
may be too small to be meaningful. Case histories
or accounts of particular events may be more useful and significant than numbers.

Outcomes Reported by Five Projects

Illustrations of evaluation used by five different
kinds of educational programs are reported. A sixth
example is the McGrath case history in the Appendix, with its specific clinical and education objectives and outcomes.

A Cancer Education Program

The ability to retrieve information about activities appears to have a direct correlation with an
administrative decision early in the project to have
a policy of continual evaluation. The Mexican-
American cancer education project is a classic example of what the Advisory Committee urges in
voicing its concern for objective measurement and
documentation of activities. As a consequence, in
the Mexican-American project:

1. Activities were not reduced to "laboratory"
experiments.

2. Evaluation activities were integrated into the ongoing project work.

3. An attempt was made to make evaluation activities educational for all participants.

4. Whenever possible, participants were involved in designing the evaluative tools.

5. The reasons for evaluation were made known.

6. The evaluation was limited.

Because of this advance preparation and policy determination, observations of factors which could hinder or improve the use of existing health resources were fed back into program planning while the project was going on. Physical and practical problems such as the consumer getting a ride to the clinic or arranging for a baby-sitter were faced, as were the broader socio-cultural problems. Changes in printed material and styles of verbal communication were some of the ways feedback altered program operation in that project.

Improving Referral and Use of Services

Can education improve accessibility to health care, continuity of care, acceptability of public health care services, primary prevention, and early intervention and treatment of disorders? Those were the tasks of the Ventura County Health Services Delivery System, and since June, 1973, a variety of successful outcomes have been reported. This project developed outreach networks within specific areas of the county. It offered a wide range of opportunities for consumers to participate in every stage of program operation.

Some of the outcomes during the first several months of operation were:

- Two thousand consumers received assistance in the procurement of needed health care, largely through local community people trained by the providers.

- Attendance at the annual Pap smear clinic tripled over previous years, due to the efforts of the community health volunteers and factory-based education sessions.

- Middle and low-income patients were accepted more readily by the private health providers.

- Thousands of dollars in unpaid medical claims were recouped for area providers.

- Private health providers became interested and involved in the instruction of low-income health consumers in good preventive dental practices.

- There was a general improvement in the acceptance of public health services by non-English-speaking consumers.

Improving Family Health

The Forty Family Pilot Study approached the improvement of health status this way: They first formulated the set of basic assumptions, described below, and then designed a program based upon these assumptions. Their assumptions are important in order to understand the scope and range of the outcomes:

- Poverty is more than a lack of economic

resources. It also includes a set of values and states of existence which exclude the poor from the opportunities offered middle-class persons.

• Citizens in the low-income group must be brought from the periphery of social living into the structure of the community. Nothing that the community does for the poor can be durably effective until the poor are a functioning part of the community.

• There is need not only for medical, educational and occupational assistance for low-income people, but especially for a system of touching the lives and attitudes of the poor so that they can take advantage of all resources available to them.

Therefore evaluation in this project consisted of measurement of progress not only in the health area, but also in the areas of housing, job development and academic education. Family development was considered a key goal—the families should become self-sustaining in a manner comfortable to them.

• 85% of the families received dental and physical examination during the first year, versus less than 5% during the year preceding the program.

• Through organized family programs, mothers became aware of nutritional aspects of meal preparation. Testing of basic health knowledge and follow-up revealed improvement.

- The number of adults receiving the General Education Diploma increased 19 percent in one year.

- All but 0.9 percent of child and adolescent participants were in school. At the beginning of the program the drop-out rate was 19 percent.

- 32.4 percent were now buying their own homes versus 20 percent a year before.

- The housing situation was somewhat improved from the previous year, although nearly half the families were still without running water.

- Average annual family income increased from $3,900 in July, 1972, to $4,960 in July, 1973.

This project illustrates a versatile health education program in which the health component became the central focus, since this resource could not be exhausted as quickly as could housing funds, for example.

Training Local Community Workers

For a number of years the concept of training local community people to provide on-site service in remote areas has been promoted without a great deal of hard data to support expansion of the idea. One of the reasons for the difficulty is the introduction of other variables in the situation which also might account for the improvement achieved. Therefore it is difficult to assess accomplishments of the community health aide or workers with regard to improvements in education, facilities, etc. However, the Alaska Native Health Service has handled the assessing of impact of the community health worker program not by attempting to isolate factors, but by describing total impact:

- "There has been an obvious improvement in health of persons in rural Alaska, probably due to many factors, but some of the improvements since the community health worker program was introduced in 1968 have been dramatic: Immunizations rates are 95 percent; no pertussis in 7 years; no measles in 8 years; no polio since 1959; in recent years diptheria only in urban areas. Pap smears were taken annually on 60 to 100 percent of eligible women as opposed to 20 percent nationally. Detection of carcinoma of the cervix in situ is increasing; invasive cervical carcinoma is declining. Infant mortality is dropping rapidly to near national levels; family planning is widely accepted; and frequency and length of stay of hospitalization is declining rapidly."

The desirability of assessing accomplishment through the choice of one strategy, such as use of community health workers, is widely acknowledged and encouraged. The inability to carry out such an assessment, however, should not be a deterrent to describing or portraying the accomplishments. Such descriptions can be helpful in following up certain aspects of the program in later stages. Such descriptions also are very useful in communicating progress as well as needs to audiences less familiar with the local situation.

Community Development

The ability of consumers to participate effectively in the planning of community health services is amply demonstrated in the Lower Rio Grande Valley program in Texas. The program shows use of community development techniques in creating opportunities for more skillful and meaningful participation in solving other problems, such as hunger, border disputes, rights to water, and justice.

Organizaciones Unidas, Inc. (O.U.) which was formed through a Comprehensive Health Planning grant, consists of 17 rural community organizations. Here are some of its achievements in the health area during the past three and one-half years:

- O.U. spearheaded the drive for two free family service clinics, each now serving over 100 patients a day.

- It brought additional needs, i.e., optical, dental, and public health services, to the attention of clinic administrators.

- It conceived and secured OEO funding for eight rural outreach centers. Information about health services and nutrition (and other subjects) was brought to the people where they live and the needs of those people were fed back to the clinics.

Methods of Recording

When considering what methods to use for recording data, it helps to make a distinction between research or demonstration projects, and service projects. Occasionally, methods useful for a research project are inappropriate for a service project. For example:

> • "We used yellow forms for reporting group meetings, pink ones for individual contacts, another color for staff meetings. God, after hassling out one meeting, to have to then sit down and write and have another meeting to go to after that. . . . Next time we tried tape recording but then the recorder had to spend time making sense out of the transcription. Evaluation might work if you were working with one group or on one little issue, but in working with 17 or 18 groups carrying multiple staff responsibilities—no way."

Techniques for recording and applying task analysis were used in some of the projects studied:

> • "Who has to know what, who has to do what, in order to say that this program is successful? What steps have to be undertaken by each category of the personnel? You can evaluate on very small numbers whether a condition is being met or not. Evaluation is a way to achieve needed mid-course correction."

Sometimes staff attitudes toward evaluation interfered with successful implementation.

> • "From the word 'Go' in our project we developed one reporting technique after another, and all failed because the staff had

other priorities and did not see of what use evaluation was. The fact that it might help someone, somehow, somewhere, some day held little attraction to them."

One technique which seemed to work satisfactorily in several projects was a series of descriptions showing how people with health problems had been guided to take advantage of health services.

In another project a monthly narrative was used to highlight workers' activities. Community workers who were comfortable with the written word wrote their reports; others reported to their supervisors verbally.

Using numbers to establish a benchmark helped another project to determine how close they were to the target. In this instance, evaluation was used to help maintain the momentum of the project and was considered an important management tool. Where anticipated objectives were used, they were set in relation to benchmarks.

Improving Evaluation

Suggestions for improvement dealt more with the need to specify the purpose of the evaluation than with methods or techniques. There are several different audiences for evaluation data, and this in itself seems to compound the problem of obtaining consistent and valid data for all the parties concerned. As others expressed it:

- "We need to ask, for whom are we doing the evaluation? What data will they accept? Scientific evaluation? Political evaluation? You really need to work with policy-makers to spell out what they want from a program."

- "Very often the evaluation is partly to satisfy the people who gave the money or to export the ideas to other areas."

A number of times the project participants discussed whether it was worth reporting experiences which did not achieve their goals. Some felt that such reporting could jeopardize future funding and support. As stated by one project participant, "The purpose of any scientific research is to see what happened, but in action-oriented projects, sometimes more important than why it failed is the fact that it took place. A later program could have been more structured from what we learned. In a new territory, it's sometimes hard to pick out the variables." In projects where no previous health service existed, this statement may be valid.

Summary

There was a general acceptance of the fact that evaluation of health education programs is possible, though difficult. It was often given a low priority. There was also general acknowledgment that more attention needs to be given to the evaluation aspects in the early planning stages of program development. Consensus was reached on the following points:

- Evaluation is conducted on a number of different levels, and the purpose of the evaluation determines the level. One purpose of evaluation is to report how funds were spent; another, to examine whether desired actions occurred efficiently; a third, to weigh the contribution of the effort against other approaches the organization can take to achieve its mission; a fourth, to examine whether this approach contributes to the problem's solution at all.

• Evaluation of research projects requires more precise control over what is to be measured, how it is to be done and how results are to be analyzed. The true value of some educational efforts cannot be measured in terms of specific immediate achievements, because the effort is directed at intangible goals that are generally accepted as valuable in our society, i.e., establishing or re-establishing feelings of self-esteem in individuals and groups.

• Regardless of the purpose or level of evaluation there should be participation in the evaluation process by those people who have been involved in the delivery of the service and by those who are served.

• There needs to be an organized way of obtaining feedback of what is actually happening in the program so that program objectives and procedures can be adjusted on the basis of information received.

• In health education where the relationship with the group being served and those serving is an evolving one, one should anticipate that original objectives and procedures will need to be re-defined and final evaluation should be based on these re-definitions.

● The educational process itself presupposes that the ultimate answer will emerge from exploration of problems and consideration of alternate solutions and therefore a firm specific outcome cannot always be promised.

● Evaluation will require the investment of time and money from the inception of the program and requires careful planning which gives attention to specificity of objectives, identification of measurement procedures, and collection of accurate baseline data.

References

1. Arnold, Mary. Criteria for Documentation and Evaluation of Cancer Education Programs, pp. 61–67. SOPHE monograph, No. 36, 1973.
2. Greene, Lawrence W. Toward Cost-Benefit Evaluations of Health Education: Some Concepts, Methods and Examples, pp. 34–65. SOPHE monograph, Vol. 2, Supplement 1, 1974.

VII. Gaining and Maintaining Support

In order to have a climate in which education can become an integral part of a health program, it is essential that policy makers and administrators develop an understanding of (1) the contributions health education can make to the achievement of health goals, and (2) the amount of staff resources needed for an organized health education endeavor. The struggle to attain this level of sustained support was reflected throughout the comments made in the program descriptions submitted, the workshop sessions and at the National Conference. In this section, the concerns expressed and suggestions offered are presented along with a brief description of new developments which hold promise for more sustained support of health education program efforts based on community needs and action, and the inclusion of education as an integral part of all health programs.

Problems Identified by Practitioners

Many programs start because money becomes available, but they fail to look ahead to what will happen when the money stops. Three-fourths of the more than 100 program descriptions submitted to the Project indicated they were funded entirely or partly by the Federal Government. Eleven of the seventeen projects reviewed in depth were so funded. Foundations and voluntary agencies were the primary sources of financial support for three others. Programs which were introduced on the basis of gradual shifting of financial support from the originating agency to a local service agency have been continued.

A realization evolved from the workshops that funders and supporters themselves have needs that must be met if support is to be continued. The Chart on Involvement indicates what limited attention was paid to these needs (See page 12.) Educational program directors are perplexed as to how one can do this effectively. Comments about this problem range from open frustration to a willingness to engage in some contrived methods which are unsettling to the program people.

● "It is important to interpret your program to funders and supporters so people are aware of your results as you go along and are ready for them. Frequently people get fired up because something is popular; unless periodic interpretation and re-interpretation occurs, the once-popular interest fades and the project will die."

● "Other people don't believe your needs and are unwilling to give money for the needs; therefore you alter what you want in order to get something someone else has, and then turn the program around to meet the need you originally saw."

Supporters, administrators and funders are often quite uninformed about the needs to be met in the development and implementation of an educational component of a program. They are unacquainted with the length of time necessary, the likelihood of a long postponed pay-off, the need for flexibility in programming and often the need to reshape objectives as new information is gained about the target population or about new, possibly more effective procedures.

- "Often the funds available are below the amount needed to obtain and sustain the educational effort needed to get the desired result."

- "We need to set goals a little differently in terms of length of time it takes to get a project off the ground when dealing with people not involved with the system. You have to build in the extra time and explain the need for it to the powers that be. It takes time to learn the community's system, too."

- "Project people must spend time—visibility time—as a physical presence in the community to let people see you, to develop a sense of trust, get to know you. When you enter a culture that is not your own, credibility time, which ranges from one month to six, is needed."

Few programs have assured long-term support. Most are conducted on a year-to-year basis. A number have been summarily ended—"Barely tooled up when we had to wind down." How can one avoid the waste of aborted program development?

- "Too-short funding, or dumping of programs, bodes ill for those who want to enter the abandoned community on another occasion. Our program, which was to run for three years, was cut off after 12 months. Can you imagine what the community will say when another university group comes around? They'll say, 'Get lost!' "

- "Community people say, 'We've been had so many times.' "

- "When the value of a new program was seen by the administrator, the cutting off of federal funds did not stop the program. He diverted other funds to keep the coordinator and outreach workers functioning."

When the documentation of outcomes includes evidence of improvement in the quality of life, some funding agencies indicate that this is irrelevant to their function.

- "When our report of a five-year follow-up was made to the government agency that funded it, they said, 'Don't bother us with that quality-of-life stuff.' "

There is need for more flexible funding and granting practices.

- "We need a grub stake to give time to involve the community in planning."

- "More grants should allow a three to six-month warm-up phase during which monies are available at a lower level than full operation. It would be more efficient, permit time for staff recruitment and training."

● "The most hideous thing about working under grants is that the end of the year comes and you have to hurry up and spend it; you can't carry money over."

Even in these demonstration projects where a new service or approach has proven its value to providers and consumers, the abrupt loss of funds terminated the program.

● "We know most of the time that funding from special projects is going to be gone. We need to plan how to make that service safe. To do this, we have any special funds allocated at the local level on a 100% basis. If a health educator is to be in that program, we talk to the local administrator and have the existing staff devote 80% of their time to the new program and 20% to general program. This proportion is adopted with new programs so that one can have continuity of staff."

Suggestions from Funders, Policy Makers, Administrators

The Project sought answers from policy makers, funders and administrators on how practitioners gain and maintain support for the educational components of health programs. These individuals were asked, What are the current policies and concerns of federal, state and local government agencies, foundations, third-party payers and others re-

garding the support of health education services?
What suggestions can be made that will answer and
satisfy them in order to bring about expanded and
continuing support for health education? What channels of communication should be used?

Here, by subject, is the advice offered by National Conference participants:

Program Support

"The Federal funding in the last three or four
years has included grants for maternal and infant
care, rodent control, family planning, lead control,
and sickle cell anemia, and all have included a
health education component. When the educational
effort is tied to a specific target or task and becomes
part of the team effort, results can be seen and the
expenditure of funds readily justified. All of these
programs have demonstrated educational results.

"At the time a grant or funding for a program is
considered, one must ask, 'Who is going to fund the
program when the grant runs out?' It is essential
that one start interpreting the need for continuing
support through the local tax-supported agency
rather than an outside agency. The people who
benefit from the program can talk directly to the
persons responsible for ending the program.

"Support for health education has tended to be
directed toward special problems. An agency needs
to develop a comprehensive staff which can add
new assignments to existing duties. Then when
more funds are available it can add more generalists
rather than specialists.

"Many make the mistake of trying to obtain
categorical grants when Federal funds are decreas-
ing while the third-party mechanism funds are in-

creasing (Medicare, Medicaid, insurance) and education has been built into the requirements or is at least permissible.

"Although the Blue Cross Board of Governors has issued a set of guidelines with regard to reimbursement for patient education which is a component of patient care, the 74 autonomous plans make their own decisions as to how and when they may wish to implement the guidelines. Educators and administrators must persuade their local plan to take this action.

"Health education cannot rely on a piecemeal application to a sympathetic foundation for basic program support. It must be built into the system of health care payment as a reimbursable service that requires continuity and an on-going organization."

Difficulty of Interpretation

"The funding of health education programs is closely tied to the concept of prevention and, like prevention, is least dramatic when it is most effective. When a problem is avoided, no crisis occurs, hence no 'miracle' is performed and the results of the effort lose visibility.

"Health education is part of public health; since it is difficult to define public health, it becomes even more difficult to define health education and its contribution. One definition is: 'Health education is not telling people what to do, but helping them to become the kinds of people who will know what to do.' "

Visibility Needed

"In view of the competition for funds the need for educators to 'sell' their program was stressed by many. In this endeavor one needs to do solid research on the interest and concerns of the funders and on what substantive information can be supplied the decision makers to give them a better understanding of the program.

"As a volunteer in the field, and as a realist, I see the need to educate the power structure, the governors and legislators, to make a commitment to health education. They must see it as a benefit, as a way of 'tooting their own horn.' You must get together with them and make them aware of how important it is.

"When an interpretation is needed at the policy level you can rarely expect a young, inexperienced person to serve. The interpreter must be a well prepared person who can make a total input but not try to dominate the decision-makers. It is often easier when one works through a new organization, since you do not have to fight the existing persons and other priorities in the system. Many professionals fail to understand the political system. A decision-maker will welcome you if you are ready with information when he needs it. Professionals usually operate on their own time table but must learn to deal with the political time table.

"The health education profession is passive. It needs a spokesman with drive, determination and logic. You can't wait to be asked. Everyone in the health decision-making process thinks he knows all about health education. They use you as a technocrat. You need advocates, and you need to present your story early in the decision-making process. You must convince them that with support for health education they will make better use of the health dollar.

"You should work with staff members of the ways and means committees of the legislative bodies. You need to infiltrate the political parties to get support for your position. Give staff assistance to state legislators. You must be on guard not to promote and protect the profession but to seek support for health education with the decision-makers. This can be done by having surrogates speak on your behalf. You need dedication, enthusiasm, and practical proof that health education does something, and that it is worth doing.

"You need public support. You should invite the press and all communication channels to help you tell your story.

"You must learn to write reports for administrators that tell your story in no more than two pages.

"There is need to look critically at what you are doing. Priorities need to be established rather than having everyone doing his own thing. There needs to be a presentation to decision-makers based on a systematic means of identifying the health needs of the target population, the resources available (including the body of knowledge about the problem), and how a specific program of action can help reduce the frequency of the health problem, that is, the personal disability which occurs, as well as the social disruptions associated with the person who has the health problem. You need to engage in a dialogue that directs itself systematically to the issues.

"Many Federal proposals have goal descriptions that do include health education. It is difficult to see how they can reach their goals of increased and more effective utilization without an educational component. This element is not recognized by many administrators. The need must be articulated by educators. There are many missed opportunities.

"The field of health education has been deprived of needed financial and administrative support. This has resulted in lack of organizational visibility and effective representation at levels where program decisions are being made. Health education should be given the same long-term support that many medical services have been given."

Approaching Foundations

"One needs to recognize that there is just as much fragmentation among foundations as among federal govermental agencies. There are very large and very small foundations in terms of staff and amounts of funds available. Many have a single theme; others are multifocused; and many are family foundations which retain members of the family as staff.

"In deciding where to seek funds, one needs to consider the generalizability of your program in terms of the size of the project and its visibility. If it is national in scope, one seeks a national foundation; if it is a community problem, then look for small, local foundations. A community effort is more likely to have success with local support sources.

"Many groups want operational support for ongoing program rather than for new programs. This is not particularly attractive for foundation funds. This is often an attempt to get matching grant funds, but many foundations aren't interested in providing operational matching funds.

"Foundations *are* interested in projects that are potentially useful beyond the particular area where the program is being developed. The idea should have potential for repetition and research. Although the programs that are almost idiosyncratic to a situation may be very important, they are not attractive to a foundation."

Project Review

"Proposals are reviewed by individual staff members and advisors prior to their getting together to exchange views. The proposal is considered on the basis of its overall intent and purpose, the methodology to be employed in carrying out the proposal. The quality of the investigator and the institution, as well as its past experience and reputation, often influence the judgment. One of the ways the staff tries to get around what might be an unfair judgment is to visit the individual to get his point of view and to see the environment.

"In reviewing projects, funders often find the following inadequacies: (1) The objectives are often not clearly, precisely and specifically outlined. (2) Proposals sound as though the project developers hope to include as much as possible, with the hope that perhaps the foundation will be interested in some segment. (3) Criteria for the appraisal or assessment of a proposal are also not included in precise and specific terms. Many if not most foundations will want the objectives and evaluation precisely defined. A grantee must avoid trying to take too big a bite and not sticking to the true potential of the project.

"Many proposals misleadingly label their programs 'demonstrations,' although it is clear that their intent is to serve a clientele, not to demonstrate the feasibility of a new approach.

"A number of the foundations interested in the health field would be quite interested in health education if the proposals were for activities quite different from what is going on at the present time."

The kinds of grant proposals that foundations look for are somewhat similiar to those that federal agencies and voluntary organizations seek, as these funders' comments show:

- "All are looking for the new approach, the innovative, fresh, invigorating idea. There aren't too many of those around."

- "We are interested in knowing what impact will the project have on the knowledge level, on health services, on the institution."

- "What amount of commitment does the agency or group proposing the grant have in the project? What are they putting in? Is there a potential that they will support the program at the end of the grant?"

- "They are concerned with researching new ideas, but they expect the applicant to have reviewed the literature to learn if the idea had been carried out 10 or 20 years ago. Many requesters do not take this step and are busy re-inventing the wheel."

- "Many small foundations do not support demonstrations."

- "Most support evaluation and are concerned with the program money that has and is being spent on ideas that have not been tested and validated."

Use of Hospital Resources

"Hospitals have been able to obtain third party

payment for health education support when the program is clearly patient education. In some cases
even out-patient services can be funded when the
insurance covers this. However, purely community
education projects at present have no visible means
of support, so the hospital must work cooperatively
with other agencies in the community in this area.
There are at least 20 examples of hospitals that view
their charter as being broad enough to include community education.

"Hospitals should look carefully at the reser-
voir of resources which they can use. Often they
have very talented employees who can be community volunteers. Many hospitals are teaching institutions, and often students have interest in broader
services to the community. Facilities are available
to share or to make available without cost."

Education Outside the Health System

"To influence the health of the population there
need to be mechanisms for education outside as
well as inside the health system, especially when
one is thinking of health care rather than medical
care. Education needs to focus on staying well and
developing healthy habits. What can be done to lead
healthier lives won't fall very heavily on the health
system, so there is a need for a mechanism outside
of the health system to promote healthful living.

"Buyers of health care need to be informed. If
they buy naively, the outcomes can be wasteful and
even disastrous. They need to learn how to make
discriminating choices. Decisions on the seeking of
care are often made when the low-income or minority person is desperate. If the resources and system
change with the advent of national health insur-

ance, then there is a greater potential for making decisions about where, when and how to seek medical care to be made in advance of being sick. The consumer needs help in making a choice on the basis of technical competencies rather than on amenities.''

Current State of Support

There is a growing recognition among funding organizations that ''an ounce of prevention is worth a pound of cure.'' Improved health education can take much of the strain off our present health care delivery system by altering the way health services are used. This concept needs further interpretation to legislators and administrators.

The Introduction contains a list of professional statements and legislative acts which have a health education focus. Half a dozen bills devoted specifically to health education support have been introduced into the Ninety-fourth Congress.

The President's Committee on Health Education stated in its 1973 report that, of the $18.2 billion allocated for health purposes, Dept. of Health, Education and Welfare estimates that it spends no more than $44 million on health education, or only about one-fifth of one percent of the total health care dollar. The Committee discovered that State and Territorial Health Departments allocate less that one-half of one percent of their budgets for health education. In 1975 the Bureau of Health Education of the Center for Disease Control, PHS, estimated in a review of all HEW activities[1] that more than $80 million is being spent on purposes related to health education by HEW agencies. There are over 30 different legislative authorities under which health education is mandated to Public Health Service organizations, encompassing such diverse areas as education on over-the-counter drugs and Indian programs.

Dr. Theodore Cooper, then Acting Assistant Secretary for Health in HEW testified[2] that ".. the central purpose of a national health education program is to build effective and appropriate health education activities into every health service delivery and resources development program, and into the public education and communications systems."

In the summary of his testimony, Dr Cooper said: "While recognizing health education of the public cannot be viewed as a panacea which will work sudden miracles, we fully recognize also that it has great potential, hitherto unrealized, for promoting better health. We believe this potential is on the road toward more effective fulfillment, and that the responsible and most effective course is to continue to build upon the initiatives now underway, both within and outside the Federal government."

The momentum is building for the support that leaders of the 17 programs stressed. The challenge now is to build on the lessons learned in the local programs and to heed the advice of the National Conference participants.

References

1. The Report of the President's Committee on Health Education, Health Services and Mental Health Administration, Dept. of Health, Education and Welfare, Jan. 1973. p. 27.

2. Cooper, Theodore: Testimony before the Subcommittee on Health, Committee on Labor and Public Welfare, U.S. Senate, 94th Session of Congress, May 7, 1975.

Conclusions

The Project has reported on the experiences of practitioners in many different and often difficult settings. Goals and aspirations of the educators were both high and broad. Their concerns encompassed improvements in access to services, reform in health care delivery, extension of community participation in health system decisions, utilization of new types of health workers, improved relationships between health care delivery and other forms of community action, and economic and social development as they relate to health conditions.

Observations and in-depth probings were made to determine what worked and where problems arose when practitioners attempted to apply accepted educational concepts and principles. These challenges inspired the imaginations and energies of many local groups as well as numerous health professionals and other leaders. This investigation brought to light past weaknesses and pointed up defects in the health system's grasp of what is involved in the educational process.

Practitioners were willing to explore their frustrations as well as their successes. This provided the Project with many insights into the gaps between theoretical concepts and their application. The Advisory Committee tried to select a wide range of anecdotal material to highlight problems and opportunities, including the need for more extensive documentation and reporting of when, where, how and why the educational process is applied, and with what success. Examples point up the need for a continuation and strengthening of existing educational approaches rather than for a drastic or dramatic re-direction.

To summarize the findings of the Project:

First, there is a need for a holistic approach to the application of the educational process to the health field. A broad spectrum of knowledge, skills and techniques must be brought to bear by many different health workers. Their talents and other available resources must be utilized to the maximum in study, assessment, planning, program implementation and evaluation that is directed toward the achievement of specific objectives.

Second, a successful educational approach requires a plan based on an analysis of the complexities present in the existing health system and the elements involved in bringing about the desired behaviors of persons who can improve the situation.

Third, resolution of many problems of poor health practices and damaging environmental conditions depends upon educating providers of health services, and legislators and regulators, as well as on managers in industry and business.

Fourth, sound educational planning takes into account the importance of providing in acceptable form the supplies, services and facilities which must be available so that people can actually adopt given practices at the point when their readiness is sufficiently high. Thus, assessment of the environment, the situation and the education of providers of facilities is fundamental in health education.

Fifth, various tools are identified for the practitioner to use in determining the many parameters of an educational problem, ways of instituting solutions, and means of assessing results along the way.

Sixth, there are many false expectations in terms of the time and resources needed to bring about individual group and community change.

Seventh, the basic theoretical concepts and principles of behavior have not been systematically applied and evaluated in many health care studies. To advance the state of the art, there must be extensive and continuing support for the research and organization of focused and effective education programs, so that anecdotal, impressionistic answers can be turned into scientifically supported judgments.

Eighth, societal decisions regarding the promotion and protection of health extend far beyond the health system. The decision as to what resources can be allocated often depends upon social opinion as to what is desirable, and on professional judgment as to what is effective and safe. The health professions need to lend their voices to seeking changes in environmental conditions which aggravate health problems.

And last, only a coordinated effort by decision-makers, institutions, providers and consumers can fulfill the potential of consumer education as it relates to health improvement.

The Committee trusts that this sharing of established knowledge and potentially useful methodology will prove relevant and rich with implications for practitioners who are engaged in education of consumers and providers. We hope that this knowledge can be combined with what is available in the vast literature of the behavioral sciences and professional fields, so that those engaged in health education can find more effective ways to improve health through the voluntary actions of consumers.

Appendix

Project Descriptions

"Tell it like it is" has been a familiar cry during the past years, yet few health education programs are reported in sufficient detail to offer guidance either to those who wish to replicate them, or to avoid the pitfalls they encountered. In an attempt to overcome this deficiency, the Project asked staff members of the 17 programs examined in depth to describe their programs as fully as possible, using a common outline.

The outline sought information about such matters as the origination of the idea itself and the length of time required for its germination. Since this part of the process of program development is seldom considered, the inexperienced administrator is usually unprepared for the very considerable expenditures of time and energy that are required to move from an idea to activity.

Program staff members who participated in the three workshop sessions expressed amazement as they examined systematically what had actually transpired in their programs. The retrospective look disclosed new strengths as well as weaknesses. Carrying out this review in the company of others who had been engaged in similar endeavors was seen as particularly valuable.

The first two summaries presented here were derived from the outline as expanded during one of the workshops. (The third project description is given with the questions used to outline it.) The outline proved useful in comparative studies of similar programs and can be helpful either as an interview or survey guide to those seeking information for themselves for individual program development or for evaluation.

Martland Hospital
Health Education Project

Martland Hospital is the city hospital for all of Newark, New Jersey, and thus is the primary health facility for inner city residents. As in most city outpatient departments, there is inadequate communication between overburdened staff and the patients. A great number of patients have not been optimally advised of their health problems or encouraged to care for their own health.

The Health Education Project (HEP), funded for three years by the Fund for New Jersey and the Hunterdon Health Fund, evolved from what was described as "an idea for improvement of health care churning in the head of one man, into a viable, ongoing organization with goals, ideas, a dynamite staff and funds." The idea was shared with representatives of community groups, nurses, physicians, administrators, security and clerical staff, all of whom helped modify and strengthen the plan. In the words of the project director, "Only by working as a group can things be restructured. Having a group involved enabled each member to act on important issues they might have been scared to act on as individuals."

An advisory group made up of members of a number of community agencies helped identify community needs and feelings. Sessions held without hospital staff present fostered open and unrestrained talk about outpatient department problems. The existence of an outside advisory group provided the basis for valuable community support for the project and its goals.

A project staff of nine was assembled. In addition to the project director, there is an assistant director, two videotape specialists, three patient expediters and two health educators.

Staff members of the hospital, the affiliated medical school and the clinic described their own past experiences with efforts to improve the clinic. This information was analyzed by the project staff for its implications for the new endeavor. Special attention was given to past successful experiences and the lessons they might have for HEP. To become acquainted with the way the clinic functioned, project staff observed actual clinic operations for three months. These observations determined how the project unfolded.

The project decided to work in just one of the 17 clinics of the outpatient department to test the validity of its plan. The metabolic clinic was selected because it served a clearly defined population; the patients required continuing care; the number of patients was of manageable size; and the staff was cooperative and open to change.

Once the metabolic clinic was selected, additional time was spent with staff to learn more about the service, to observe its performance and to discuss the project in greater detail. Patients' attitudes and knowledge were determined through observation and survey. A questionnaire was used to determine how much patients knew about their medical problems. It was the exceptional patient who knew what he or she was being treated for, or why.

The results of the fact-finding phase showed that a number of organizational changes needed to be made in clinic activities to facilitate or, indeed, to make possible improved patient-staff interaction. For example, on any given day 15 percent of patient charts were not available in the clinic. Staff and patients lost valuable time until these were located. Sixty percent of laboratory results were not recorded in patient records. Patients had failed to follow the verbal directions to go for laboratory work in 34 percent of these instances; the remaining absences of laboratory records were attributed to departmental difficulties. Both patients and professionals were frustrated by these deficiencies.

There was no staff continuity for the clinics—nor did staff know until the days they reported which patients were expected. Block appointments made long waits inevitable for patients. Few patients knew what clinic they were attending.

Consideration of these findings by the clinic and project staff resulted in the following steps to establish clear routines and responsibility for staff and patients:

1. The professional staff re-arranged schedules to provide greater continuity of nursing and physician service.

2. Block appointments were replaced by individual appointments.

3. Patient care expediters from the Health Education Project staff were assigned to the clinic to answer questions and to check on charts and routines a day *before* each clinic session.

4. The expediters distributed pamphlets and showed patients videotapes (described later) produced by the project.

5. A laboratory instruction sheet in both English and Spanish was prepared to guide patients in obtaining the nesessary tests in other parts of the hospital.

6. A patient information card, not previously used, was prepared listing the patient's name, address and phone number, and containing the name of the physician and the medicines prescribed.

7. Changed procedures in the metabolic clinic were interpreted to staff and patients verbally and with the aid of printed instruction sheets.

Materials Developed

A number of information materials have been produced by the project, both to explain individual health care instructions, and to inform patients about other health issues affecting their lives.

The goal of the project is to bring about more effective and meaningful interaction between patients and health care services. To accomplish this, services in the out-patient department were restructured and improved by:

1. developing better communications between patients and staff;

2. establishing clear routines and responsibilities for both staff and patients;

3. providing patients with specific information on how to use the clinics;

4. developing health information to meet patients' needs;

5. providing health information developed by the project to community groups for use in their own settings.

Carrying Out the Project

Capitalizing upon the appeal of television, especially to those who read with difficulty, videotapes seven to ten minutes long were produced by the HEP staff. Community people and users of the clinics appeared on the tapes, explaining and dramatizing subjects such as how the outpatient department works, ways of preventing accidents around the home, and the hazards of lead paint poisoning. Additional videotapes on medicine-taking, immunization, and the meaning of comprehensive health care and how to get it are in production. Care is taken that the actors, scenes, manner of speaking and music used all are familiar to residents of Newark.

The project staff, with the help of clinic personnel, developed a series of simple pamphlets which describe how the outpatient department works and which include a map of its physical layout. A patients' newsletter and a newsletter for clinic staff is published. These materials are distributed from a "Patient Aid Station," a small oasis in the general waiting area of the outpatient department. This station, staffed by the HEP patient expediters or community volunteers, is a place for information, for patients complaints to be heard and for referrals. Additional such stations are planned for other locations.

Results

1. There has been a consistently favorable change in the number of appointments kept. The appointment system change is understood and followed. Patients know how to get in touch with the clinic if they must cancel their appointments. Missed appointments now are followed up through use of the patient card and the efforts of the patient expediters.

2. Greater continuity of care exists, as patients are more apt to see the same physician on their return visits.

3. Retrieval of laboratory information has improved greatly. Where formerly only 40 percent of results were available when needed, now 97 percent are in place. Procedural change and more careful directions to patients have brought this about.

4. Patients have assumed a more active role in obtaining care by seeking out the staff when they don't feel they have satisfactory answers. Access to the videotapes and pamphlet materials, plus the help of the patient expediters, has helped build the confidence of the consumers.

Materials and programs developed in the project are being used with community groups as planned. The results of the project have been visible and positive. It has been a fruitful educational program for both staff and patients with a potential for extension to the entire outpatient service.

McGrath Demonstration Project

In 1957 a demonstration study, headquartered in McGrath, Alaska, was inaugurated in six isolated villages in rural Alaska. Its purpose was to determine what practical measures could be found to lower the prevalence of upper respiratory infection and to prevent complications. A two-pronged approach, clinical and educational, was used.

The plan called for initial surveys to assess the physical status of all children under 17 years of age and to measure the level of health knowledge and practices of their families. This was to be followed by a period of intensive education and medical care, with a final reassessment of health status, knowledge, and practices to evaluate the amount of change, if any. The first phase, the baseline survey, was completed in September and October, 1957.

The second phase consisted of an intensive educational program conducted by all members of the team and a medical care program undertaken by the project physician and two public health nurses. These clinical phases were based on the needs revealed by the baseline surveys. Phase two extended from late fall of 1957 to September 1959.

The third phase of the project was the resurvey period in the fall of 1959.

The fourth phase extended through several months of 1960, when reports were completed and final tabulations and analyses of the data were made.

Information collected included household census data, demographic information, socio-economic and nutritional data, prevalence of selected eye, ear, nose and throat conditions, and information on health knowledge, practices, and habits.

Results

Improvement in physicial status as measured by healed tympanic membranes, lowered incidence of newly ruptured drums, and decreased chronic middle ear infection (otitis media) was achieved at a significantly measureable level. Substantial changes in health knowledge and in many health practices occurred. It was found that it was possible, in the space of less than two years, to lower the incidence of some of the disabling complications of upper respiratory infection, and to change the level of health knowledge and some of the health practices related to understanding and care of these conditions. Here is a summary of the findings and specific experiences relating to them.

Clinical Changes in 485 Native Children:

1. Chronic otitis media was reduced from a rate of 12.6 per hundred to 6.6; over 65% of the cases, prestudy and new, were treated and healed.

2. Rate of perforated tympanic membranes dropped from 18.4 per hundred in the baseline survey to 13.2 at final examination. A cure rate of 72.8% was realized on cases developing during the project period.

3. Chronic otitis media rate was 17.1 in infants born before the project started and zero in infants born during the two-year span of the project. The rate of perforated membranes was 27.6 in pre-project babies and 12.0 in the newborns.

Health Practice and Knowledge Changes:

1. Sponge bathing as a means of reducing fever was used by 63.2% of the families in 1959, in contrast to only 29.9% in 1957.

2. Thermometers were available to 74% of the families and 40% were using them in 1959, in contrast to 1957 when only 9.1% of the families had them.

3. Steam inhalations as a treatment increased, with 47.2% of the families using steam in 1959 in comparison to 31.2% in 1957.

Three Types of Objectives of the Educational Program

In the McGrath project the major subject areas needing team attention were quite obvious from the survey data. Four principal criteria were used in developing the education content and objectives. These were:

1. Health conditions needing attention, as revealed by the baseline physical examinations.

2. What people needed to know and do in order to prevent these conditions.

3. What people already knew and did and what they still needed to learn, as indicated by the baseline data.

4. What people probably would and could do.

It was found, for example, that unlike the situation elsewhere in many areas of Alaska, eye pathology was not a common condition in the six villages. Therefore, concentration on information about eye disease was considered unnecessary. On the other hand, the frequency of draining ears and hearing loss indicated the need for emphasis on these problems.

The primary objective was to help people improve their health, especially as it related to upper respiratory infections. It was considered basic that the people in the villages should learn to assume responsibility for early recognition and treatment of these infections, and to seek expert help when needed. The desired outcomes of the teaching program were specific:

1. Educationally, it was desired that people should *know* and *understand:*

A. The germ theory of disease and concepts related to transmission and modes of spread, especially of upper respiratory infection and its complications.

B. Early signs and symptoms of upper respiratory illness, especially middle ear infections and how to recognize them.

C. How to distinguish between conditions that can be treated by the family and village health aides and those which require professional medical care.

D. How the ear works, its relationship to the nasopharyngeal area, and the need for early care in order to prevent hearing loss.

E. The importance of early and adequate treatment.

F. The importance of explicitly following instructions for recommended treatment and medications.

G. The relationship of good general health to resisting disease, especially: good sanitation and personal hygiene, sound nutrition, adequate clothing for the weather, and good rest habits.

2. Behaviorally it was desired that people understand the need for, and learn when and how to carry out, the following home care techniques:

A. Use of the thermometer (when, why, and how).

B. Use of sponge bathing as an aid to fever reduction.

C. Use of steam inhalations to help relieve congestion and respiratory distress.

D. Use of nose drops to keep the eustachian tube open.

3. It was desired that people make proper use of medications available in the village and know how to seek needed additional assistance from the local health aides, public health nurses, and Native Health Hospitals.

4. The team also hoped to develop the following positive attitudes toward maintenance of health and prevention of upper respiratory illness:

A. They wanted to develop the attitude that draining ears are not inevitable and that action on the part of the family is necessary.

B. They wanted people to feel that upper respiratory infections should never be considered insignificant as far as need for treatment is concerned.

C. They wanted people to feel that the practices being advocated are socially acceptable and economically worthwhile and should be carried out in fishing and hunting camps as well as at home.

In the educational phase of the project, it was found that more learning took place when (a) teaching was done in intimate family-size groups; (b) teaching centered around existing clinical problems and relevant situations; and (c) the teaching methods and aids used by each health worker were ones with which she felt comfortable.

Unique Characteristics

Two aspects of the McGrath study appear to be unique: (1) an intensive medical care *and* treatment program carried on *simultaneously* with intensive education in those things that people must do for themselves; (2) the capability to change techniques and methods in accord with the findings uncovered in the baseline studies, in order to reinforce the teaching of people how to take care of themselves.

There is a tendency to separate, if not isolate, medical care and treatment from education. In the McGrath project, people learned from the experience of the clinical examination and treatment in an organized, planned manner. Learning takes place when information is relevant and meaningful. Acceptance of the new information and belief in its validity appears to have taken place with long-lasting results, according to present day clinical impressions of the McGrath area. The youngsters of this study are the new parents of today.

Educational Observations

Two different types of examples illustrate the problem of cultural value differences. The first is based on interviewing on an individual basis; the second, on a community socio-economic basis.

In the phase of interviewing in regard to health practices, there was considerable semantic confusion. To a question such as "When people have fever, do they need special foods?" respondents frequently wanted to know whether soup, water, juice, or Koolade were special foods. The word "when" gave frequent difficulty, since the respondents' connotations did not seem to include "for what reasons" or "on what occasions." Therefore confusion was expressed when staff asked about *when* children should wash their hands or *when* the temperature should be taken.

The second illustration of cultural value differences is related to the attempt to gather socio-economic data to determine the correlation between the socio-economic factors and the presence of disease. The data had to be discarded. The main problem was that there was no way to set up a standard for measuring or converting non-cash income into cash values. Furthermore, there was no way to determine the quantity of various food items. A barrel in one village would not be equivalent to a barrel in another. Food preservation practices also varied from locality to locality and from family to family within a village and could not be given a dollar value.

Moose and other game had a wide range of weights in terms of available and edible meat. People were understandably reluctant to list out-of-season game they had caught. Redemptive values for items such as fur could not be determined, since they were based not on the number obtained, but on the quality and place of redemption. Payment received from a trader might be applied to past and current accounts so that it was impossible to estimate income for any one year. Fish preserved for use by family and dogs was never weighed.

These are examples of the kinds of differences which must be taken into account in the design of a meaningful educational program.

VISTA Bi-lingual Health Aides

HEALTH EDUCATION PROJECT DESCRIPTION

Name of Project:
VISTA Bi-Lingual Health Aides

Name of Individual Reporting:
Christine Ling, Health Education Officer,
Hawaii State Department of Health
P. O. Box 3378
Honolulu, Hawaii 96801, Tel. (808) 548-5888

Sponsoring Agency:
Health Education Office
Hawaii State Department of Health

Source of Funds:
ACTION (formed on July 1, 1971) to coordinate Federal
volunteer service programs of which VISTA (Volunteers
in Service to America) is one of six.

Budget:
VISTA estimates direct cost of support of each volunteer
is $8,600 per year. The sponsoring agency provides costs
in kind—i.e., desk space, supervision, paper supplies,
equipment and other tools necessary.

Date Project Began:
July 24, 1973

Expected Life Span of Project or Completion Date:
One year from start with probable extension to an additional three years.

I. *Brief History*

A. *Where did the idea for this project originate?*

The seed for the project was planted by an ACTION consultant who had been the State Director of Public Education. He called on the Health Education Officer on January 26, 1973, and in an informal discussion suggested that volunteers might be effective in extending the work of the Health Education Office to working with the "disadvantaged."

B. *What steps were taken to gather information about implementing the idea?*

Informal calls were made on several program managers within the Hawaii State Department of Health and, in this preliminary discussion, the Communicable Disease Division expressed the most interest. They reported rising tuberculosis rates in Hawaii were caused by persons newly arriving in the State. Within the Health Education Office a sub-program for immigrants is in operation, headed by a bilingual public health educator. In the cold statistics of the Health Department, data was readily available on the pressing health problems of the immigrants from the South Pacific and Southeast Asia. Information on health problems, as seen by the agencies and the immigrants themselves, was not as readily available.

The public health educator, Dr. Herita Agmata, was extremely interested in obtaining volunteers, as she had felt aides were needed to deal directly with the various groups in their own neighborhoods.

C. *Who was involved in its development?*

The Health Education Officer pursued the idea with the ACTION director in Honolulu who, after considerable discussion, agreed to modify the basic idea to health as a goal rather than a more catholic approach of helping meet basic needs which might not have been health-related. The necessary clearance was obtained through the Director of Health, the Dept. of Health Business Office, and the Governor, as there was a freeze in program expansion.

D. *What changes, if any, took place in discussions or negotiations with others during its development?*

During March, the Health Education Officer took the leadership in convening interested private and governmental groups in the geographical area where newly-arriving immigrants were settling, for an early involvement in problem identification, goal setting, objective development, work plans and evaluation measures. The VISTA staff provided direct assistance with the write-up of the project proposal. A decentralization of operations was agreed to.

E. *How long did it take to get the program underway?*

During March and April, the five agencies who committed themselves to the project worked on goals, objectives, job descriptions. The completed project proposal took four months to develop.

F. *What resources of staff, facilities, etc., were available?*

The Health Education Office of the State Department of Health provided the supporting services, guided by the locally-based ACTION office.

G. *To what specific problems does this project address itself?*

The project is directed at controlling tuberculosis, other communicable diseases, parasites, and in securing available health services for newcomers.

H. *What was done to authenticate the problem?*

Hard data already available in Department of Health records.

I. *What records were kept of the program's implementation?*

The project proposal became the guideline for the implementation of the project. VISTA asked for an evaluation of the project according to VISTA guidelines.

II. *What was the overall goal of the project?*

To have bilingual health aides establish contact with newly-arriving immigrants to assist them with problems relating to tuberculosis and to help them gain access to available community health services.

III. *What were the specific objectives?*

Specific objectives were developed by the five participating agencies and varied according to the agency's primary orientation.

IV. *What is the target population?*

Newly-arriving immigrants from the Philippines, Korea, China, and Samoa.

V. *What methods were used to involve the target population?*

1. Utilizing immigrants with training in

health or in health-related fields (college graduates) and with bilingual ability.

Because immigrants are reluctant to utilize the services available in the State for fear of becoming a public charge and thus being deportable, it is necessary to communicate and to reach the target group in order to gain their confidence.

In order to communicate and to reach the target population, it was necessary to use persons who speak the same language as immigrants and who could be visible in the area where the immigrants are predominantly located and where services are needed. The outreach workers are immigrants who know the culture and the problems of immigrants.

Generally, health is not the primary concern of immigrants. They are more concerned with employment, housing, money, etc. Therefore, in order to gain the confidence of immigrants, the aides need to help them with their pressing problems.

2. Involving people living in the same area.

3. Placing in selected community centers and clinics workers who are responsible to the supervisors in these centers and clinics.

4. Contacting immigrants
    a) by door to door visits;
    b) through referrals (schools, churches, public and private agencies, community organizations, hospitals, etc.)
    c) by follow-up of specific problem cases.

5. Mass media (radio, newspaper, TV).

VI. *What specific actions were carried out?*
1. Recruitment of aides.
2. Training of aides (pre- and in-service training) in the following:
    a) Knowledge of health care system in Hawaii, i.e., public health laws, rules and

regulations, individual and community responsibilities.

b) Communication skills: two-way communication; how to interview, how to interpret, how to write reports.

c) Content knowledge: Immigration laws and amendments, tuberculosis, basic hygiene, communicable diseases, epidemiology of parasites, nutrition, maternal and child health, etc.

d) Community facilities and services: How to utilize available resources and what to expect of agencies and professionals, i.e., physicians, public health nurses, social workers, teachers, etc.

e) Knowledge of medical regimes: How to take medications and to follow instructions.

3. Placement of aides in agencies:
   a) Immigrant Centers
   b) Clinics
4. Contact of immigrants by aides.
5. Follow-up of cases by aides.
6. Neighborhood meetings.
7. Community meetings (youth groups, mothers groups, church groups, etc.).
8. Workshops.
9. Health fairs.
10. Development of health information materials.
11. Development of record-keeping of contacts made with immigrant families.
12. Development of guidelines for information desired for individual and family health status.

VII. *What are the outcomes of the program?*

1. From August 13, 1973 to January 31, 1974, the aides (5) contacted 2,757 immigrants and en-

couraged approximately 65% to obtain medical and other needed services.

2. Aides arranged neighborhood meetings, community meetings and workshops, and assisted in health fairs to reach target groups.

3. Health information in the Samoan, Korean and Philippino languages was developed and distributed.

4. Aides followed up on cases referred by agencies, professionals, hospitals and schools.

VIII. *How did you verify these outcomes?*

1. Monthly reports by aides.

2. Checking the health assessment forms.

3. Interviews with immigrant families known to the aides.

4. Talking to health professionals, social workers and school personnel about the value of the services of the aides.

IX. *What aspects of the program were not completed as planned?*

The original plan was to hire 10 aides. In August, 1973 only seven started with the program. After two months, three resigned. Because of financial needs, the three who resigned had to find other jobs with better pay. In September, two aides were hired. In December, one aide resigned after passing the RN board examinations. In March, 1974, four aides were hired. At present, there are nine aides.

X. *Did any benefits result that were not anticipated?*

In spite of the resignations and shifting of the volunteers, in six months they were able to reach more than half of the expected number of immigrants to be contacted and have helped approximately 65 percent of the immigrants obtain the needed services.

XI. *What circumstances in your opinion have influenced why this program took the shape it did?*

 1. Concentration of the immigrants in certain areas of the State helped the aides in reaching them and proving to the immigrants that use of services and acceptance of assistance did not result in deportation.

 2. Continuous follow-up of the immigrant families by the aides.

 3. Establishment of rapport between the aides and the immigrant families.

 4. Cooperation and coordination of services of agencies and help of the Health Education Office staff.

 5. Availability of funds through VISTA.

 6. Continuous influx of immigrants.

 7. Enthusiasm of aides who can communicate with immigrants and who have the same background and culture and who have an appreciation of the problems of recent immigrants.

XII. *What evaluation was carried out, either by self-evaluation or by others?*

 1. Records were reviewed of:

  a) Total number of immigrants contacted.

  b) Total number of immigrants assisted by aides to obtain needed services.

  c) Total number of services utilized by immigrants.

 2. By interviews or questionnaires to determine:

  a) Attitudes of recipient families about the value of the services rendered by aides.

  b) Attitudes of professional health, welfare, school and other agency personnel.

  c) Health practices followed by survey for better health, i.e., complete immunizations, nutrition, etc.

XIII. *As a result of this experience, what future plans do you have?*

The program is in its infancy. With only seven months experience and a favorable result, we are asking VISTA for an expansion to four more neighbor islands in a rural setting, with resident health educators to supervise the aides.

XIV. *What has been the long-range impact of your program?*

No data yet available.

XV. *Describe any constraints you experienced at any stage in the development of your project.*

A fiscal constraint was placed on the Health Education Office. No additional funds would be provided.

XVI. *What advice would you give to someone trying to carry out a similar program?*

1. Involve Early All Persons who might be interested. The directors of the agencies were brought in from the beginning, but we had to backtrack to include staff persons.

2. Clear the Decks: In Hawaii, with constraints placed on the expenditure of public funds because of a tight financial situation, clearance had to be obtained from the Director of Health, the Department of Health's Business Office, and the State Department of Budget and Finance, and the Governor. VISTA was constantly given new deadlines, so there was some anxiety in obtaining the letters of clearance.

3. Allow Sufficient Time: The project development involved more time than anticipated. There was some confusion in VISTA requirements for training, and with the obvious need to provide our own orientation to the Hawaii system. Supervision of the volunteers took anywhere

from 40 to 60 percent of staff's time. The project director recruited, organized the training, and developed the interview evaluation forms.

4. Get Expert Help in Developing Evaluation Instruments: My feeling is that we will need to re-evaluate our instruments. The over-all goal is to assist with tuberculosis control, but the helping relationships should be measured, too.

5. Anticipate Some Built-In Problems in an enterprise involving several agencies: VISTA, as a governmental agency, has certain goals, expectations, etc., but in a changing Federal role new guidelines and goals were established. The interpretation by VISTA volunteers who staffed the local office fluctuated. Calls had to be made to San Francisco to clarify procedural matters involving the recruitment, training, etc. of the volunteers. The recruitment was a joint responsibility and the prospective volunteer was interviewed by VISTA, the Health Department, and the agency staff where he or she was to be placed.

XVII. *Special Materials Developed:*
1. Health Assessment Form.
2. Family/Individual Record Form.
3. Health information in Samoan, Chinese, Korean and Philippino.

Steps in Program Planning

The following outline presents proposed steps in program planning for effective health education efforts. Examples of how to proceed in documenting information, applying criteria, and determining the evaluation procedures are offered by the Committee to assist the health education practitioner. Readers may also wish to consider the planning approach used by Weed* in analyzing the problem-oriented medical record (POMR).

I. Collect Information About the Health Conditions of the Target Population. Organize the recording of the information obtained. The example given below applies to ways in which the information for a health education program for a local neighborhood health center might be organized:

    A. Information on Personal Health Practices.
    HOW OBTAINED:
      1. Interviews with household samples.
      2. Interviews with community workers, e.g., extension health workers from county health dept; welfare workers; teachers.
      3. Community reports from other agencies, e.g., Office of Equal Opportunity, social surveys by universities or community groups, etc.
    HOW DOCUMENTED:
      1. Overall arrangements and direction by staff

---

* Weed, Laurence L. Medical Record, Medical Education and Patient Care. Press of Case Western Reserve Univ. (distributed by Yearbook Medical Publications, Inc., 35 East Wacker Drive, Chicago, Ill., 1971.)

health educator in consultation with sociologist, social service survey staff and health personnel to design interview questionnaire and to use existing data. Indigenous persons may be hired to collect new data.

B. Use of Existing Health Services

HOW OBTAINED

1. Review morbidity and mortality statistics.
2. Review health dept. records.
3. Review outpatient and emergency room records of hospitals, neighborhood health center records, welfare records, Medicaid, etc.
4. Interview private practitioners (M.D.)
5. Self-reporting as part of interviews in part (1.) above.

HOW DOCUMENTED

1. Health educator in collaboration, whenever possible, with a marketing staff person and medical staff.

C. Following of Medical Advice

HOW OBTAINED

1. Interview a small sample, a random selection of patients in a variety of settings: family health center, clinics, hospital out-patients, private physicians, to determine what advice is followed and what advice is not followed and why.

HOW DOCUMENTED

1. Registered nurse and licensed practical nurse in the settings selected plus health dept. public health nurse follow-up with patients. Health educator designs interview form with staff from agency.

D. Participation in Program Development

HOW OBTAINED

1. Analysis of response to community meetings, expressions of interest or program suggestions to Board members, staff, etc. Volunteer activity.

HOW DOCUMENTED

1. Health educator responsible for data, obtain-

ing information from all staff. Records attendance and participation by age, sex, geographic location and occupation.

E. Related Information

HOW OBTAINED

    1. School reports in health and social problems.

    2. Court reports.

    3. Literacy reports and census tract data.

HOW DOCUMENTED

    1. Medical and nursing staff, social worker, health educator.

II. Apply Criteria to Each Problem Identified Above, Then Select One Problem for Analysis. The following illustrate criteria which might be applied to problem:

A. Level of interest and concern of the service population and the providers of care. Will the program have a measurable effect on the illness pattern of the community? Did organizations find ways to collect information from a cross-section of the consumers in the target population?

B. Availability, now or potentially, of materials for problem analysis and evaluation.

C. Amount of disability/death caused by the problem (both in numbers and severity).

D. Relative contribution to general welfare of population served.

E. Availability of control measures (technically and economically feasible).

F. Availability of resources to carry out education program.

G. Acceptability of control measures.

H. Possibilities of change through education.

    1. Degrees of stimulation/motivation needed to accomplish change.

    2. Ease of identifying and reaching the target population.

    3. Does the program (problem) lend itself to innovative educational approaches?

I. Compatibility with existing health programs and social and environmental conditions.

J. Potential consequences of the program.

1. Will the program lead to other actions that will make for a continuing consumer involvement in an improvement of health?

2. Will it raise the level of health concern among the target population?

3. Will it affect the way the consumers relate to the health system?

4. Will it increase their understanding of how to manage their own health?

K. What is the potential for progress toward resolving the problem or accomplishment of the outcomes within the time allotted to the project?

L. How applicable would this program be to other poverty areas in the United States?

III. Analyze Selected Problem in Terms of:

A. Probable causes and contributing factors (e.g., misunderstanding, unfavorable attitudes, cultural conflicts, bad fears, inconvenience, costs).

B. Probable barriers to bringing about needed changes.

C. Past attempts at education concerning this problem.

1. Resources and methods used.
2. Problems encountered.
3. Results.

D. Experiences, attitudes, and skills of consumer group concerning education (e.g., what sources are most likely to be trusted, what methods accepted, reading level?)

E. Organizations and individuals that should be involved in program development, e.g., representing:

1. Consumers
2. Providers
3. Educators
4. Communications media
5. Behavioral scientists
6. Possible funding groups
7. Other

IV. Develop Objectives in Specific Measurable Terms That Can Be Used In Evaluating Outcomes; e.g., in relation to changes in consumers' and providers' understanding, attitudes, skills and behavior.

V. Develop Criteria For Use In Selecting Educational Approaches.
    A. Potential for bringing about desired changes.
    B. Acceptability to consumers and providers.
    C. Availability of needed personnel, equipment, facilities, and money.
    D. See II. above.

VI. Select An Educational Approach or Combination After Applying Criteria To Alternatives Such As:
    A. Group discussion.
    B. Role playing or simulation games.
    C. Videotape playback.
    D. Audiovisuals for presentation to groups or individuals.
    E. Programmed instruction.
    F. Individual counseling.
    G. Mass media.
    H. Use of educational prescription, especially to guide team education of patients.
    I. Use of indigenous aides, e.g., for counseling or advocacy in homes or clinics, and for feedback from the consumers.

VII. Develop a Work Program and Budget for Implementing the Selected Educational Approach.
    A. Delineate specific activities designed to achieve objectives. Show anticipated starting and ending time for each activity. For example, one activity might be re-education methods for clinic personnel.

A timetable covering an eighteen-month span is shown below as an example.

Operations

	N D J F M A M J J A S O N D J F M A
Select Problems	‾‾‾‾
Analyze Problems	‾‾‾‾‾
Set Objectives	‾‾
Select Approaches	‾
Develop Work Program	‾
Staff Recruitment	‾‾‾‾‾
Staff Training	‾‾‾‾‾
Implementation	‾‾‾‾‾‾‾‾‾‾‾
Review Progress	X X X X X X

B. Determine kinds of skills needed to carry out activities, then decide on staffing pattern and responsibilities.

C. Develp budget, keeping cost/effectiveness in mind.

D. Determine organizations and individuals to contact for follow-on commitments for paid and volunteer personnel, committee involvement, equipment, facilities, money, etc.

E. Develop plans for evaluation, e.g.:

    1. Baseline data.

    2. Periodic process review to determine if principles of effective educational program development are being used.

    3. Periodic reviews of progress toward achievement of objectives.

VIII. Determine Specific Roles, Responsibilities, and Relationships of All Advisory and Technical Committees, Task Forces and Consultants.

Workshop Participants

In addition to those listed below, Advisory Committee members chaired the workshops, and all members participated in the National Conference.

Ms. Susan Goodfriend, Coordinator
Institute of Public Affairs
801 Second Avenue
New York, NY 10017
ROOSEVELT HOSPITAL (NYC) HEALTH EDUCATION PROJECT

Ms. Marcia Heller, Instructor in Health Administration
Columbia University School of Public Health & Administrative Medicine
21 Audubon Avenue
New York, NY 10032
PROGRAM OF CONTINUING EDUCATION

Peter Lazes, Ph.D., Project Director
Health Education Project
Martland Medical Center
65 Bergen Street
Newark, NJ 07107
MARTLAND HOSPITAL HEALTH EDUCATION PROJECT

George A. Lentz, M.D., Medical Director
Community Pediatric Center, W. Redwood Street
University of Maryland
Baltimore, MD. 21201
UNIVERSITY OF MARYLAND COOPERATIVE EXTENSION SERVICE HEALTH EDUCATION PROJECT

William Lloyd, M.D., Medical Director
Martin Luther King Health Center
3674 Third Avenue
Bronx, NY 10456

Ms. Ellen Manser, Advocacy Team Director
Family Service Association of America
44 East 23 Street
New York, NY 10010
PROJECT ENABLE

Ms. Evelyn Miller, Project Director
ACE Local Action Program
1 Commerce Blvd.
N. Amityville, NY 11726
SUFFOLK COUNTY ASSOCIATION HEALTH
    GUIDE PROGRAM

Ms. Rita Pacheco, Chief, Public Health Educators Section
Office of Public Health Education
New York State Dept. of Health
84 Holland Avenue
Albany, NY 12208
NEW YORK STATE HEALTH GUIDES PROJECT

Mr. Hayden Reiter, Health Education
Community Pediatric Center, W. Redwood Street
University of Maryland
Baltimore, MD 21201
UNIVERSITY OF MARYLAND COOPERATIVE EX-
    TENSION SERVICE HEALTH EDUCATION
    PROJECT

San Francisco Workshop
April 24–25, 1974

Mr. Adelbert L. Campbell, Coordinator
Area IX, California Regional Medical Program
7700 Edgewater Drive
Oakland, CA 94621

Volna Curry, Ed.D., Project Director
American Cancer Society, Los Angeles County Branch
1550 W. 8th Street
Los Angeles, CA 90017
MEXICAN-AMERICAN CANCER EDUCATION
  PROJECT

Mayhew Derryberry, Ph.D.
1401 Walnut Street
Berkeley, CA 94709

Walter Johnson, M.D., Medical Director
Alaska Native Medical Center
Box 7-741
Anchorage, AK 99510
COMMUNITY HEALTH AIDE TRAINING
  PROGRAM

Ms. Christine Ling, Health Education Officer
Hawaii State Department of Health
Box 3378
Honolulu, HI 96801
VISTA BI-LINGUAL HEALTH AIDES

Ms. Patricia Mail, Public Health Educator
CHR Coordinator, IHS Western Washington Service
  Unit
USPHS-IHS
1212 S. Judkins
Seattle, WA 98144
COMMUNITY HEALTH REPRESENTATIVE

Ms. Sarah Mazelis
1043 Dolores Street
San Francisco, CA 94110

Mr. Thomas M. O'Brien, Project Director
3147 Loma Vista Road
Ventura, CA 93003
VENTURA COUNTY HEALTH SERVICE DELIV-
ERY SYSTEM

Harriet Schirmer, M.D., Project Director
Wrangell, AK 99929
McGRATH PROJECT

Columbus, Ohio, Workshop
May 29–31, 1974

Ms. Betsy Baker, Health Educator
The District Health Department
Box 191
Chapel Hill, NC 27514
BYNUM MILLS PROJECT

Amanda A. Beck, Ph.D.
Office of Aging
Michigan Offices of Services to the Aging
1026 E. Michigan Avenue
Lansing, MI 48912
CONSUMER SUPPORT PROJECT

Ms. Eleanor Eaton
Community Relations Division
American Friends Service Committee
160 N. 15th Street
Philadelphia, PA 19102
TEXAS CONSUMER EDUCATION PROJECT

Mr. Jose Fuentes
9001 La Barranca, N.E.
Albuquerque, NM 87111

Mr. Domingo Gonzales, Chairman
Texas Consumer Education Committee
2804 Tulipan
Brownsville, TX 78520
TEXAS CONSUMER EDUCATION PROJECT

Ms. Linda J. Hayman, Health Education Consultant
Indiana State Board of Health
1330 W. Michigan Street
Indianapolis, IN 46206
FORTY FAMILY PROJECT

Ms. Elizabeth Lee, Staff Associate
Division of Education
American Hospital Association
840 N. Lake Shore Drive
Chicago, IL 60611

Mr. Richard Panzironi, Director of Health Education
Family Health Center
117 W. Paterson
Kalamazoo, MI 49007

Ms. Judy Van Roekel, R.N., Public Health Nurse
The District Health Department
Box 191
Chapel Hill, NC 27514
BYNUM MILLS PROJECT

Ms. Janice H. Williams, Acting Director of Education
Atlanta Southside Comprehensive Health Center
1039 Ridge Avenue, SW
Atlanta, GA 30315
PRACTICAL NURSE TRAINING FOR NEW PROFES-
SIONALS

Conference Participants

**National Health Education Conference
Augusta, Michigan, Oct. 27–29, 1974**

Amanda A. Beck, Ph.D.
Office of Aging
Michigan Offices of Services to the Aging
Lansing, MI

Mr. Berkeley Bennett, Executive Vice President
National Council of Health Care Services
Washington, D. C.

Leroy Burney, M.D., President
Milbank Memorial Fund
New York, NY

Mr. Adelbert Campbell, Coordinator, Area IX
California Regional Medical Program
Oakland, CA

Vernal Cave, M.D., President
National Medical Association
Washington, D. C.

Mr. Robert M. Cunningham, Consultant
Blue Cross Association
Chicago, IL

Effie O. Ellis, M.D.
Special Assistant for Health Services
American Medical Association
Chicago, IL

Paul M. Ellwood, Jr., M.D., President
InterStudy
Minneapolis, MN

Ms. Barbara Farmer
Evaluation Unit Consultant
Albert Einstein College of Medicine
Bronx, NY

Ms. Florence Fiori, Director
Division of Resource Development, HEW, PHS, Region
II
New York, NY

Mr. Herbert Gatzke, Director
Bureau of Manpower & Education
American Hospital Association
Chicago, IL

Mr. Domingo Gonzales
Chairman, Texas Consumer Education Committee
Church & Society Commission
Harlingen, TX

Mr. John K. Iglehart
Senior Editor (Health)
National Journal Reports
Washington, D. C.

Mr. Charles T. Lanigan, Vice President
Metropolitan Life Insurance Company
New York, NY

Peter Lazes, Ph.D., Project Director
Health Education Program
Martland Medical Center
Newark, NJ

Mr. Edward Levin, Chairman
Health Education of the Public Committee of the Governor's State Health Policy Council
Milwaukee, WI

Ms. Christine Ling
Health Education Officer
Hawaii State Department of Health
Honolulu, HI

Ms. Rose Marie Love, President
National Health Consumers
Chicago, IL

Mr. Donald J. Merwin, Project Director
Developmental Project on a National Center for Health
    Education
National Health Council, Inc.
New York, NY

Ms. Evelyn Miller
Project Director, ACE Local Action Program
N. Amityville, NY

George E. Miller, M.D.
Director, Center for Educational Development
University of Illinois College of Medicine
Chicago, IL

William E. Mosher, M.D., Commissioner
Erie County Health Dept.
Buffalo, NY

Ms. Lorna Otto
Community Health Representative
Division of Indian Health
Mt. Pleasant, MI

Alberta Parker, M.D.
Clinical Professor of Community Medicine
University of California School of Medicine
Berkeley, CA

Selected Bibliography

Bennis, Warren G., Benne, Kenneth D., and Chin, Robert. The Planning of Change: Readings in the Applied Behavioral Sciences. Holt, Rinehart and Winston, New York, 1961.

The scientific basis of the processes involved in bringing about change in the individual, group and community are examined. Part III, which discusses the dynamics of the influence process, is particularly relevant to persons working in health education programs. This section included excellent guidance for the practitioner by presenting the application of theory as discussed by Leland Bradfor, Kurt Lewin, Herbert Kelman, Edgar Schein, Cora DuBois, Alvin Zander, and Anselm Strauss.

Cantor, Nathaniel. The Teaching-Learning Process. Holt, Rinehart and Winston, New York, 1953.

Anyone engaged in the helping process will find this basic text on the teaching-learning process valuable for the perceptive discussion of present perceptions of education and the need for the teacher to understand the personal process of change. This work laid the ground for Miller's later text on Teaching and Learning in Medical Schools.

Freeman, Harold E., Levine, Sol, and Reeder, Leo G.

Handbook of Medical Sociology, Prentice-Hall, Inc.,
Englewood Cliffs, New Jersey, 1963.

Three chapters are particularly relevant for community health workers who wish to develop a framework for analyzing the community structure and to
introduce change. They are: "The Community and
Health Organizations"; "Public Health in the Community"; and "Health Action in Cross Cultural Perspective" which cites concepts which apply equally
well to the sub-groups within U.S. communities.

Health Education Monographs, Society for Public Health
Education, Inc., Charles B. Slack, Inc., Thorofare,
New Jersey.

> Vol. I No. 13 Alvin Zander. "Influencing People
> in Face to Face Setting: Research
> Findings and Their Application."
>
> No. 27 Marjorie Young. "Review of Re-
> search and Studies on Health Edu-
> cation Practice" (1961–66); "Pro-
> gram Planning and Evaluation."
>
> No. 32 Marvin D. Strauss (ed.). "Con-
> sumer Participation in Health Plan-
> ning."
>
> No. 35 Marjorie Young. "Review of Re-
> search and Studies on Health Ed-
> ucation and Related Aspects of
> Family Planning" (1967–71);
> Communication, Program Planning
> and Evaluation."
>
> Vol. II No. 4 Marshall H. Becker (ed.). "The
> Health Belief Model and Personal
> Health Behavior."
>
> Vol. II No. 1 Carol D'Onofrio and Virginia Li
> Wang. "Cooperative Rural Health
> Education."

Houle, Cyril O. The Design of Education. Jossey Bass, Inc., England, 1972.

This is a blueprint for planning, setting up, implementing, and evaluating adult education programs. Houle's system is in two parts: adult learning situations are classified into 11 categories; second, he puts the plan into action by providing step-by-step procedures—a basic framework or model, applicable to all categories. The two parts make up an efficient new system which combines modern theory and practical procedures.

Knowles, Malcolm S. The Modern Practice of Adult Education: Andragogy Versus Pedagogy. Association Press, New York, 1970.

This book is divided into three parts: Part 1 explores the differences between pedagogy and adult or andragogy learning and the meaning of the differences to the development of unique adult education methodology. Part 2 is a systems approach to educational program planning and operation and Part 3 presents tested management procedures for courses, workshops, institutes, and other types of educational activities.

Knutson, Andie L. The Individual, Society, and Health Behavior. Russell Sage Foundation, New York, 1965.

The author states the book presents "a description of man as a unified social being . . . the constructs employed to interpret man's health-related actions have been examined from different points of view and illustrated in a variety of ways." Of particular interest to the health education practitioner is the theoretical underpinning for perception, motivation, values, attitudes, and beliefs which are then applied to learning, the communication process, and obtaining health action.

Krech, David, Crutchfield, Richard S., and Ballachey, Egerton, L. Individual in Society: A Textbook of Social Psychology. McGraw-Hill, New York, 1962.

An introduction to social psychology with the use of the interpersonal behavior event as the unit of analysis. The authors look at the individual and what goes on within the person as well as looking at the social habitat of the individual. Combines theoretical concepts from social psychology, social anthropology, and sociology. Has an extensive discussion of cognitive theory, motivation, social attitudes, language and communication, culture, groups and organizations, leadership and group change, the effective group, and the individual and the group.

Lippitt, Ronald, Watson, Jeanne, and Westley, Bruce. The Dynamics of Planned Change: A Comparative Study of Principles and Techniques. Harcourt, Brace and Company, Inc., New York, 1958.

Although an older publication, this is a well focuseo book on the process of planned change and the various roles of the change agent. The topics covered include diagnostic orientations, motivation of the client system, initiation and phases of planned change, and transfer and stabilization of change.

Nyswander, Dorothy. International Symposium: Papers on Theoretical Issues in Health Education, September 27–28, 1974. University of California, Berkeley, California.
A selection of 16 papers on key issues in health education written from the practitioners' and researchers' viewpoints. It is the most recent review of practice and leads for future research practice in the field.

Paul, Benjamin D. Health, Culture, and Community. Russell Sage Foundation, New York, 1955.

A series of community case studies, each dealing with a concrete health situation, are presented to illustrate successes and failures in how a community went about trying to solve a health problem. Thus the book presents what happens rather than what ought to happen. The 16 case studies focus primarily on rural settings in other countries; however, the basic concepts are equally applicable in the U.S. The author's comments in the introduction and final chapter on review of concepts and contents help the reader translate specific examples into general principles which can be examined and applied to work in any community.

Warren, Roland L. Perspectives on the American Community: A Book of Readings. Rand McNally and Company, Chicago, 1966.

This book contains both the traditional approaches to studying a community and illustrations of some of the processes of planned change as they relate to community problems. The author presents the fundamental conceptualization of what a community is and important ways of thinking about a community from the points of view of sociologists, anthropologists, political scientists, and urbanologists. He also presents how to study a community in terms of structure and function, interaction, and the dynamic aspects of the social processes.

Watson, Goodwin (ed). Concepts for Social Change. National Training Laboratories, National Education Association, Washington, D.C., 1967.

The book contains the working papers developed to give direction to the Cooperative Project for Educational Development. The authors present concepts about organizational development, or self-renewal as a form of planned change; an analysis of resistance to change; collaborative action-inquiry; and the use of social research to improve social practice. Finally, Matthew Miles and Dale Lake discuss the self-renewal model as it applies in school systems.

Wise, Harold, Beckhard, Richard, Rubin, Irwin, and Kyte, Aileen. Making Health Teams Work. Ballinger Publishing Company, Cambridge, Massachusetts, 1974.

The authors set forth the values implicit in health team operation and offer suggestions on how to cope with the problems health workers face in delivering comprehensive health care. The book records the development of a team approach to family-centered health care at the Dr. Martin Luther King, Jr. Health Center. It contains a look at the overall administrative structure necessary for the team method, the roles, decision making, power distribution, and staff education. The analysis builds on the Lewian Life space model.